BRINGING IT ALL TOGETHER

BRINGING IT ALL TOGETHER

The Chiropractic Perspective for Better Structural and Functional Health

Dr. Jim M. Weber

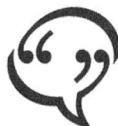

YouSpeakIt
PUBLISHING
*The Easy Way
to Get Your Book
Done Right*™

To all those seeking a course to regain their health.

*I also wish to dedicate this book to my wife,
who has inspired me to reach for my goals with both
hands. Thank you, Pauline!*

PRAISE FOR
BRINGING IT ALL TOGETHER

"Dr. Weber provides a clear, concise, and tremendously useful outline for how modern preventative medicine is really about each individual taking control of their own health and realizing the full spectrum of proper preventative healthcare that is available to them."

— Jared C. Kneebone
Apex Energetics
Territory Representative
Northern California Region

"Jim has always been an inspiration to me. In *Bringing It All Together,* he explains in a fun, yet straightforward way how the biomechanics of the body align to allow for healing. He also explains how life stresses can cause misalignment and lead to poor health. As he goes through the different parts of the body, he shows how each system not only relates to each other system, but also how our digestion, our hormones, the regulation of inflammation, our nervous system function and so much more are all related to our body's alignment. Jim and I believe that the more we understand about how the body operates, we then have a roadmap of what can be done to assist the body into a state of health. Chiropractic care is one of the major adjunct therapies that I recommend to my clients when they are undertaking a nutrition program as proper alignment allows for better and faster healing."

—Linda Clark, MA, CNC,
Owner, Operator of Universal Wellness Associates
Adjunct Professor at John F. Kennedy University,
Speaker and Author and Creator
of Detox 360°™ Program and Gluten-Free Life™

"As a Sports Medicine and Functional Medicine Chiropractor for over 35 years, I recognize that patients having information about their conditions is critical to them following through with care. This book does an excellent job of providing important information. Dr. Weber has a unique knack for making complicated information very clear and understandable for everyone.

"As a patient, I recognize that there is more to being a great doctor than just 'book smarts'. Dr. Weber has the compassion and 'the touch' necessary to be both. He has knowledge, experience and skills that set him apart from the rest of his profession. I highly recommend his book and his care."

—H. A. Bud Walker, DC, CCSP
Owner, BeWellSacto

Contents

Acknowledgments

Many people have influenced the content and the writing of this book. Many of them won't be listed here, and for that, I offer my deepest apologies. I am grateful to you all.

A special thanks, first and foremost, to my wife, Pauline, who always pushes me to be at my best. Thanks, of course, to my family, who are always supporting me in every way.

To my aikido sensei, Wayne Wallace, who has been instrumental in helping me understand structural integrity.

To Dr. David Peterson, who has been a good friend and mentor and has helped to show me the complexity of the human structure and many of its intricate parts.

To Dr. Mary Unger-Boyd, another mentor and teacher, who was extremely influential in helping me become the doctor that I am.

A great big thank you goes out to my patients! Without you, this phenomenal art of healing that we call chiropractic wouldn't be what it is. Thank you to the thousands of patients who we have helped and learned from and the many more to come. It is through you that we can do our part in healing the world.

Thank you to everyone for being a part of my world.

Introduction

Why is it that pain will be sharp one day and then general the next?

Have you ever wanted to know why your muscles are so tight even though you stretch?

Why is it that so many issues, for example fatigue, brain fog, and digestive issues, wax and wane throughout the day?

This book will address these questions and more. I touch on many of the topics that have frustrated my own patients over the years. It was only through working with my patients and studying rigorously that I was able to discover the best path to helping them achieve health solutions.

Chiropractic is a relatively new form of healing compared to other arts like acupuncture, aromatherapy, homeopathy, and so many more. Manipulative therapy has been documented as early as 400 BCE.[1] Today's therapies included under manipulation mainly constitute osteopathy and chiropractic. Traditional therapists who practiced the art of spinal manipulation were called bone-setters,

---

1 Pettman, Erland. "History of Manipulative Therapy." Journal of Manual and Manipulative Therapy, 2007. doi: 10.1179/106698107790819873

and these practitioners have been traced back to Egypt, China, Indonesia, and many of the countries around the Mediterranean.

In chiropractic school, we are taught that structural care will assist the body in healing. However, it wasn't until after a couple of years in practice that I really began to challenge that dogma. My biggest question was, "Is structural health more important than functional health?"

Structural health is the premise that chiropractic was founded upon: by having a balanced spine, you will be healthy. Functional health deals with the inter-workings of our bodily organ systems, including the blood and lymph systems.

After all, in chiropractic school we are taught that the spine is our lifeline due to the nervous system. I asked: *What about every other system that helps our nervous system work, like the blood and all its nutritional components? How about the lymphatic system and its ability to get rid of all our cellular metabolic waste?* So many systems have been left in the dark. So, I am going to attempt to shine some light and walk through some important concepts to help you better understand the art of chiropractic.

In the chapters that follow, I describe:

- How structure and function are interwoven
- How inflammation influences both structure and function
- How key structures play a role in our overall health
- The role of digestion
- The importance of our mindset and attitude toward our own health

Along the way, I discuss possible solutions and daily habits to improve your odds for a long, healthy life.

My name is Dr. Jim Weber. I am a Sacro-Occipital Technic (SOT®) doctor of chiropractic. I live in Sacramento, California, where I have a thriving practice with my beautiful wife, Dr. Pauline Asahara, who specializes in pediatrics. Since I began my study of human anatomy and physiology, I have been fixated on the notion that the body has the ability to heal itself.

As I began seeing patients, I knew that Dr. Major Bertrand DeJarnette was right. I paraphrase him when I say: *Anatomy and physiology and neurology don't change between patients; they only adapt to the individual's own stressors.* It was this certainty that led me to read books like *Gray's Anatomy* and *Guyton and Hall Textbook of Medical Physiology* (Saunders: Elsevier, multiple editions), along with many others. I knew that if I gained a deep understanding of what normal was, there was a greater chance I could identify the abnormal.

One of my teachers said it best: *Finding the problem is the hard part.*

After many successful cases and others from which I learned the most, I knew I had to spread the word about the common theme I was seeing among my patients. Many had no idea what I was doing to help them or why it helped. This is why I decided to put this book together.

Once you identify what the problem is, the solution often becomes evident. However, you must have the knowledge to understand what you are seeing.

This book is different from most because it describes applying chiropractic work to change lives. It has been my life's work to translate medical terms — X-ray reports, lab findings, and medical textbooks — for patients in a way that shows them the best options to change their own health. After almost a decade in practice, I had to get my thoughts onto paper and into as many hands as possible.

Much of what I know I have learned through treating patients who, after having seen countless healthcare practitioners, found their way into our office and —

finally — found their answers to a better way of health. Those patients have taught me so much. To honor them, I want to pass on their experiences to others who may benefit from them. Please enjoy.

It is my hope that by reading this book, you will see that *taking initiative* to prevent disease provides a better outcome when compared to those who are more *reactive*. These days, our healthcare system is in serious trouble, and the average person is just waiting for ill health to find them. Chronic disease, in the form of dementia, diabetes, ADD/ADHD, celiac disease, fibromyalgia, and many others, is overwhelming our communities. It only leaves you one of two options: act today and take the initiative to improve your health, or wait for a disease process to take hold.

> *By the year 2040, an estimated 78 million adults, about 25 percent of our population, will have a doctor diagnose an arthritic problem, compared with the 54 million adults diagnosed by 2015.*[2]
>
> ~ Centers for Disease Control and Prevention

---

2 "Arthritis-Related Statistics." Centers for Disease Control and Prevention. July 18, 2018. cdc.gov/arthritis/data_statistics/arthritis-related-stats.htm.

Let's take a second and break down the word arthritis. The origin of arthritis comes from the Greek word *arthron,* which means joint. The suffix *-itis* is used by numerous terms to denote inflammation. So, arthritis literally translates to *joint inflammation.*

Question for you: If we take away the inflammation in the joint, does the arthritis go away? This concept will be discussed later in greater detail.

This book will open your eyes to many aspects of health that you intuitively already know but from which you have been led astray. The simple fact is that our bodies have this amazing ability to heal if given the right opportunity and time.

After reading this book, I hope you become more interested in the benefits of functional chiropractic care. It is my intention to help readers to understand what a doctor of chiropractic can offer patients, not just in structural correction, but also for long-term wellness.

CHAPTER ONE

Better Biomechanics From Day One

BETTER STRUCTURAL ALIGNMENT IMPROVES BODY FUNCTION

> *There cannot be health until there is emotional, physiological, endocrine, secretory, absorption, elimination, and proper anatomical balance of all cellular parts.*
>
> ~ Dr. M. B. DeJarnette

We are all striving for wellness and a good, healthy body. In 2009, I began practicing as a chiropractor. I have discovered, through my work with each patient, how rectifying the body's structure, along with improving the function of the organ systems, promotes wellness and long-lasting health.

Alignment Promotes Healthy Flow Through Blood and Lymph Vessels

When you align the musculoskeletal structure of the body, you promote the best flow of oxygen, nutrients, and metabolic waste through arteries, veins, and lymphatics. As Dr. M. B. DeJarnette explains:

> In wellness, the body is a collection of intelligent cellular units. Each cell communicates to each other by chemical messengers that the majority of them travel in the blood. Each cell is dependent on the neighboring cell. There cannot be health until there is emotional, physiological, endocrine, secretory, absorption, elimination, and proper anatomical balance of all cellular parts.

This is key to having well-rounded health in our body, the wellness we are striving to achieve.

As a chiropractor, I always look at the structural aspects, or the biomechanics.

The basic fundamentals of chiropractic are:

- The sacrum and the ilium, which make up the pelvis
- The spine
- The cranium, made of the facial bones and the cranial vault — twenty-two bones total

Most importantly, I check the blood and lymph. As I view these aspects, I am aware that the structural integrity of the human body depends on the mechanical perfection of each part. The body will function well only to the extent of that mechanical perfection.

However, I also keep in mind that the chemical stressors we constantly deal with in our lives ultimately cause the breakdown of the structural system. This breakdown can then clog, impede, and impair the blood flow and lymphatic flow, which causes congestion, and this congestion will result in a decline in health and wellness.

Keep in mind that muscles move bones. Bones are held together by ligaments. As inflammation begins to impair the ligaments, the breakdown of the system will follow. Inflammation is simply our immune system alerting our body of danger, calling in cellular reinforcements to heal. In acute or sudden scenarios, this is extremely beneficial and necessary. However, over long periods of time, this can be problematic. We will discuss inflammation and the impairments it creates later in more detail.

Muscle Tone Promotes Flow of Oxygen and Nutrients to Organ Systems

When inflammation breaks down the tissues of ligaments, the joints lose their integrity and begin to separate. The resulting misalignment is a chiropractic problem called *subluxation*. However, most chiropractors love to jam it together via an adjustment. The chiropractic adjustment may be done by manual correction or by tool or by machine. This adjustment should not be feared, but understood. To have long-lasting health and good muscle tone, as a chiropractor I want to help you prevent or minimize subluxation.

You can think of it this way: As ligaments become stretched and impaired, the muscles must work harder. A muscle's sole job is to contract and relax. If we are able to heal the ligament, this means the muscle can do its job.

As the inflammation process continues, the muscles around all joints begin to become more spasmodic, more in spasm, or in greater contraction. For instance, if you feel that one muscle of your back is usually tighter than the others, this may indicate an imbalanced pelvis. This imbalanced contraction will cause impaired blood flow as well as an impaired lymphatic system.

The lymphatic system is your body's sewer system. When flow is impaired, it becomes clogged with wastes. Exercise and movement help with the elimination of waste; however, proper body function through chiropractic care significantly helps balance the system.

The inflammatory process will increase muscle spasms in acute circumstances, which can be useful. However, most adults experience chronic inflammation, which ultimately leads to poor muscle tone and a loss of strength. As we age, we often think that growing weaker is just a fact of old age. In fact, an inflammatory process is often the cause of these changes in our bodies as we age. This process can cause loss of muscle tone and other symptoms that directly affect your health and wellness.

Breathe Properly and Lower Your Risk of Organ Congestion

> One of the most helpful things you can do to help calm anxiety and other types of fears and stress responses is abdominal breathing.

The pelvis includes the sacrum and the ilium, and the joint between them is your *sacroiliac joint*. This is a location that commonly requires chiropractic treatment. One of the major muscle groups that helps hold the pelvis together is the *iliopsoas* or *psoas muscle*. The iliopsoas muscle attaches to all the lumbar vertebrae, the pelvic bones, and the diaphragm. The diaphragm and its three leaves are a continuation of the iliopsoas muscle.

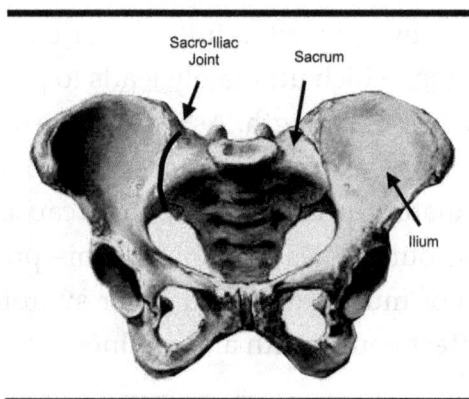

When the pelvis becomes imbalanced, the psoas muscle — usually one side only — will contract. The opposite side will contract to try to counterbalance it. However, all the digestive organs are positioned between the diaphragm and the pelvis. The distortion pattern that causes the muscles to contract on one side versus the other ultimately causes an imbalance through the entire system. The imbalance decreases the space between the diaphragm and the pelvis, leading to spastic organs. Common symptoms, such as gastric esophageal reflux disease (GERD), heartburn, spastic colon, and constipation are caused by this constant muscle imbalance. These can be chronic issues for adults, but children may also have symptoms, such as gastric reflux in babies, because of this same phenomenon.

One of the strategies that helps resolve these issues is chiropractic therapy. In addition, it may be helpful to address faulty digestive chemistry, which is addressed in the next section.

Proper breathing is an aspect of wellness that is often overlooked, but it is of great importance in helping to support health. If you watch a baby breathe, the baby's abdomen will expand with each breath; this is the proper, healthy way to breathe. However, abdominal breathing is uncommon in adults today; instead, many adults are *chest breathers*. Abdominal breathing is one of the most helpful things you can do to calm anxiety and other types of fear and stress responses. In addition, abdominal breathing helps massage the area to achieve lymphatic decongestion for the internal organs.

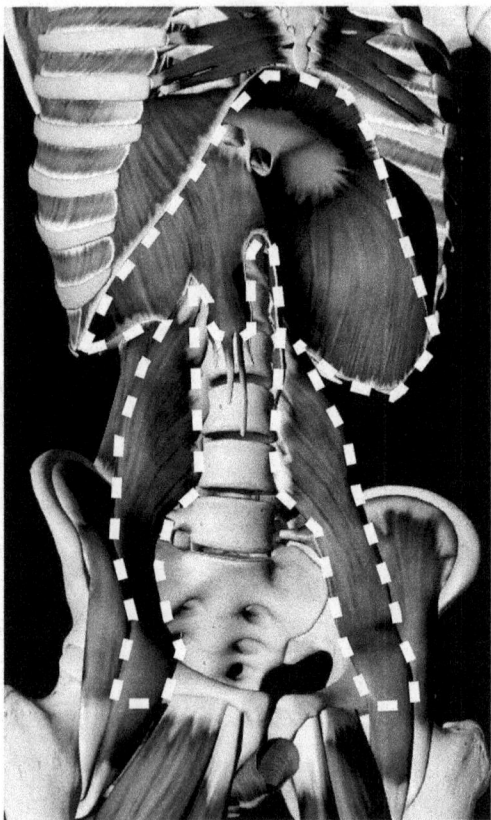

The dotted line illustrates the ilio-psoas muscle. Notice its
connection between the diaphragm and pelvis

A BALANCED PELVIS AND CRANIUM LEAD TO OPTIMAL HEALTH

Some of the most common things that we see in a chiropractic office are neck pain and low back pain. Correcting the imbalances of these structures is described in this chapter as keys to good health and proper and long-lasting wellness.

When fetuses develop before birth, multiple systems become integrated to work as one. The first system to develop is the nervous system. This nervous system is encased in bone, from the head all the way down to our pelvis. It makes sense that the entire nervous system is protected by bone; it is so important. The description below explains how important this sensitive structure is.

Sacrum: The Powerhouse for the Digestive Organs

The pelvis is made up of the sacrum, which is the triangular portion of the pelvis; and the ilium, which is the uppermost and largest part of the hipbone. This structure is crucial because this is the basis of the body's entire structural system.

The sacrum is the most important component of lower digestive health because approximately the lower third of your gastrointestinal system depends on the part of the nervous system that routes through your sacrum. Gastrointestinal and uterine-related ailments, such as menstrual cramps, commonly cause low back pain originating in the sacrum. Uterine health and presentation is crucial not just for menstruating women but also for proper fetal development during pregnancy. If the soon to be mom's sacrum is *subluxated* (dislocated) or *torsioned* (twisted), there is a good chance the uterus will be torqued, and the baby has a higher risk of a breech presentation.

The sacral plexus, which is the nervous system tissue in the sacrum, is the distribution and reception mechanism for the lower third of the bowel. Normal sacral motion acts like a rocking chair to promote proper bowel function, proper immune function, and most importantly, relaxation and calming. As babies, we were soothed by being rocked. The sacrum is designed to rock back and forth as we move. This rocking promotes and governs proper parasympathetic function, which is what supports relaxation, repair, and digestion. In another section, we will talk about how autonomic function is crucial in this aspect.

The sacrum is only half the equation; both the cranium and sacrum must be balanced for good health. The next section will discuss the importance of *temporomandibular joint* (TMJ) health.

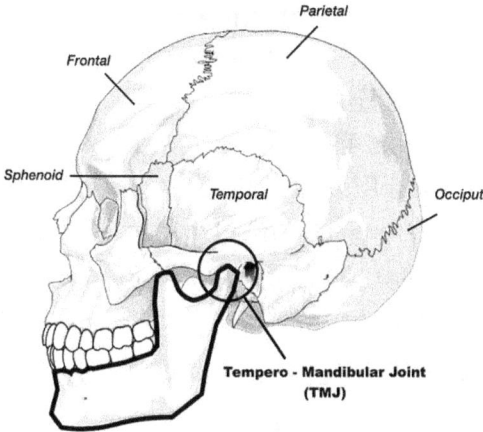

Parietal
Frontal
Sphenoid
Temporal
Occiput
Tempero - Mandibular Joint
(TMJ)

Proper TMJ Function Is the Way to Good Digestive Health

The TMJ is the only freely moving cranial bone; the rest of the skull is only capable of micro motions by means of sutures. The TMJ helps the movement of the entire cranium, which supports blood and lymph flow throughout the entire cranium. However, the most important aspect of the TMJ is that it is the lifeline to the digestive tract. If you don't have proper TMJ function, you won't have proper digestive chemistry.

The *gastrointestinal* (GI) tract is approximately thirty feet long and extends all the way from your mouth to your anus. It is made up of the oral cavity, the esophagus, the stomach, the gallbladder, the pancreas, the small intestine, and the large intestine. The function of the GI tract, or *gut,* is to break down food into small molecules that the body can absorb to feed our cells. This highly complex system absorbs nutrients and eliminates toxins through a number of physical barriers, chemical processes, and immune processes. Each part of the GI tract has a specialized job in the breakdown and absorption of food.

Dr. DeJarnette, one of my mentors and a successful researcher, provided priceless amounts of data to help the health and well-being of humankind. One of the gold nuggets he uncovered during his research was that anytime a jaw issue or *temperomandibular joint dysfunction* (TMJ) is found, the muscles and ligaments create a pulling to one side, which causes the esophagus to pull or torque as well. This pull on the esophagus affects the tissue pull directly into the stomach. This tissue pull stresses the stomach and disrupts normal physiological mechanisms like stomach acid production, intrinsic factor, and lipase activity. In addition, the painful chewing that occurs with TMJ will cause a person to avoid foods that require more chewing. A lot of times, people who chew poorly will swallow food prematurely, before it is properly broken down. The poorly chewed food will cause more stress for our digestive organs, which can cause putrefaction—rotting of the food.

The TMJ has four main muscle connections to the head, including the *temporalis muscle,* which helps us close our jaw while we are chewing. Temporomandibular dysfunction causes the muscle to spasm; it may have difficulty relaxing, and in some cases, can't completely relax at all. Someone with this dysfunction grinds upper and lower teeth at night because of gravitational forces on the body when they are lying horizontally. Teeth-grinding causes an abnormal wear pattern, leading to an abnormal bite. The abnormal bite will perpetuate further TMJ issues, which may lead to greater digestive health issues and an imbalanced pelvis.

Proper jaw activity is vital from the time we are very young. The mechanics involved in the nursing process for an infant, in fact, are very important to infant development. Proper nursing requires using both lips and latching properly while holding the nipple. Improperly designed bottle nipples may push the lips apart; as a result, there is no need to hold on to the nipple while latching. The natural suckling motion created by the infant extracts milk and activates the bone-forming centers in the *maxilla,* which is the upper jaw. Without this jaw activity, digestion and enzyme activity throughout the gut is minimized.

Balance Leads to Good Autonomic Function and Good Health

> The cranium governs the upper two-thirds of the digestive function, and the lower sacrum controls the lower third.

Many times, a person with an imbalanced pelvis will also have an imbalanced TMJ. As we are painting a picture of what a balanced pelvis does for our digestive health and what a balanced cranium does for our digestive health, it is important that we look at both ends of the spectrum. What's a picture if it's only half-complete?

Now that we have painted a picture of how the cranium governs the upper two-thirds of the digestive function and the lower sacrum controls the lower third, it is time to look at the overall autonomic function. A balanced pelvis and a balanced cranium will lead to good autonomic function, to promote the best health.

Activated by **Exercise & Stress**	Autonomic Nervous System		Activated by **Meditations & Rest**

Sympathetic	**Parasympathetic**

• Fight & Flight • Increases Heart Rate • Pushes blood into arms, legs and head • Pushes blood away from digestive organs • Adrenal glands activate release of catecholamines	• Rest & Digest • Decreases Heart Rate • Serotonin & GABA stimulate parasympathetic function • Improves blood flow to digestive organs

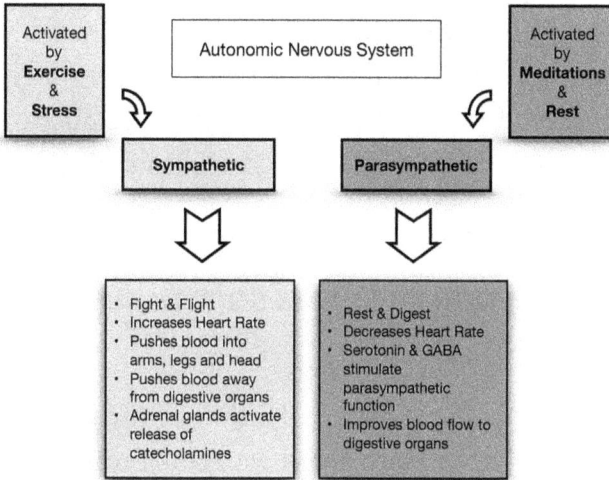

The *autonomic system* includes both your sympathetic and your parasympathetic systems. The *sympathetic system* is your fight-or-flight response system. Your *parasympathetic system* is your rest/relax/digest system. Most people have a sympathetic dominant issue or parasympathetic withdrawal issue, meaning the stress pushes us past the ability to rest, repair, and digest efficiently. This pushes our body into survival mode, which results in our body using its own resources for survival. Over time, our body will use its own proteins stored in its muscles, ligaments, and bones to sustain our daily existence. This is one of the reasons why we lose strength as we age, why we lose bone integrity, and so much more.

For example, obesity and tiredness, combined with an inability to think clearly, are big issues for a lot of people. These symptoms may result from poor autonomic function that is caused by a structural or biochemical imbalance in the cranium and the pelvic structures.

INFLAMMATION DESTROYS SOFT TISSUE

In our toxic world, inflammation is common. Inflammation is the result of either trauma, infection, or exposure to toxins. These aspects of inflammation over time are termed *chronic inflammation*. This can happen without our awareness and ultimately destroys our structural health. Inflammation resulting from exposure to toxins will break down the structures supporting our health, and it can happen without our awareness. It is the goal of this section to explain how inflammation destroys soft tissue.

Inflammatory Proteins Degrade Structural Proteins

A lot of people think inflammation only happens when something is swollen. Actually, inflammation is a natural part of our healing process. When you get cut, that cut turns red, it swells, and it becomes tender to touch. These aspects of inflammation are a part of healing.

However, chronic inflammation can be a serious problem.

It can result in a multitude of symptoms, like:

- Swelling
- Arthritis
- Fatigue
- Brain fog
- Bloating and gas
- Skin issues, such as acne and eczema
- Weight gain
- Moodiness
- Sleep issues
- Irritability
- Tinnitus

A standard blood test can check for inflammation by identifying markers such as homocysteine, ferritin, C-reactive protein, decreased cholesterol — usually below 150 — a high-density lipoprotein (HDL) level below 50, as well as more specialized inflammatory markers. If markers are abnormal in the blood test results, it means that inflammation is destroying soft tissue as described previously in this chapter. For example, looking at levels of the first marker, homocysteine, allows us to assess the potential breakdown of structural proteins. Specifically, proteoglycans and other collagen-forming proteins in our muscles and ligaments are at risk of breakdown if homocysteine levels are high.

As these inflammatory proteins continue to degrade, not only do they break down muscles and ligaments, but they also attack organs and unbind the connections of the nervous system, ultimately affecting overall health and wellness.

Inflammation Drives Up Cortisol and Insulin

Inflammation tends to drive up both cortisol and insulin. Insulin is an anabolic hormone that allows glucose to enter our cells efficiently. Cortisol is a catabolic hormone that allows for the proper breakdown of stored glucose, or glycogen levels. Inflammation in acute circumstances is beneficial because it is taking defensive actions to support allergen or pathogen elimination, immune efficiency, and tissue healing.

Blood sugar issues, which may be connected to inflammation, interfere with hormones, energy levels, and sleep patterns. Chronic blood sugar imbalance and consistently high insulin levels often lead to diabetes. High glucose levels in people will drive up insulin levels, which subsequently will affect cortisol levels.

Chronic cortisol elevations, which will be discussed in the next section, will cause thinning of the gastrointestinal lining. Chronic cortisol issues also impair our immune system and several other systems that negatively impact our energy, sleep, and mood — to name three symptoms of a long list.

Insulin and cortisol stimulate each other. Whenever someone has a high insulin level, they also tend to have a high cortisol level, which will exaggerate stress responses. More stress responses increase insulin, which, in turn, raises blood sugar. It becomes a vicious cycle, which needs to be broken before a healthy state can be restored.

Inflammation Thins the Lining of the Gut

As described in in the previous section, inflammation causes increased cortisol and insulin. The effects of inflammation on the gastrointestinal lining are many. With acute stress, a higher level of cortisol occurs, which leads to the immune system in the gastrointestinal tract being suppressed or lowered. So, when a high level of cortisol occurs, that leads to a less efficient gut immune system. This eventually causes a decrease in protection of beneficial gut flora, which ultimately causes a decrease in the amount of stomach acid the body produces. A decrease in stomach acid prevents the body from having a strong protective mechanism to combat pathogenic microbes that may enter our body through food or other sources. With decreased stomach acid comes a higher risk of bacterial overgrowth, which will lead to gas and bloating.

As stomach acid decreases, the body also loses its digestive sequencing. As explained previously, the digestive process starts in the mouth and ends in the anus. Digestive processing has a sequencing effect as well. As you chew, you make stomach acid. As you make stomach acid, you have greater enzyme release and better absorption of foods. Chronic stress combined with long-term insulin and high amounts of cortisol will break down the mucus lining, which then causes complete loss of beneficial microbes. These circumstances leave the gastrointestinal tract open to leaky gut or more inflammation.

Chronic stress may result in a sympathetic-dominance condition, causing a lack of parasympathetic function to stimulate neurotransmitters, such as serotonin or GABA (gamma aminobutyric acid), which are key to promoting healthy sleep, rest, and digestion— elements of the parasympathetic system. Sympathetic dominance places the body in a higher state of fight-or-flight.

Chronic stress causes a breakdown of the mucosal lining because, as the cortisol is being released in acute stages, it eventually causes the adrenal system to be exhausted. The adrenal system is our energy reservoir, which helped our ancestors to escape tigers, bears, or other predators. Today, our adrenal glands are our fight-or-flight system, which, for most people, is activated way too much. This chronic activation is what leads to immune system suppression, gastrointestinal issues, sleep disturbances, skin problems, and many other health issues that cause loss of health and wellness.

One of the best things we can do for ourselves is to lower inflammation. This will ultimately cause our bodies to respond better to health therapy, whether it takes the form of massage, nutrition, exercise, or other therapies. Inflammation impedes many efforts to regain one's health — diets, detoxification, exercise routines, or whatever. Without lowering inflammation, none of these efforts to return to health will be beneficial. The cause of the body's breakdown will persist.

I have been to many different chiropractors over the years and was mostly told that it would take a few days after each adjustment to feel the benefits, and I would need to continue a weekly regimen with the doctor. When I saw Jim for the first time, I knew this was different. How he could pinpoint issues and resolve them was incredible! He would adjust me and have me walk around. If anything was still off, he would have me get back on the table until it was gone. I've never experienced that before, and I am more than grateful to have found his practice. I could not recommend Quantum Chiropractics more highly.

L. Halldorf, Real Estate Agent
Sacramento, CA

CHAPTER TWO

Health Starts in the Gut

PROPER DIGESTIVE CHEMISTRY IS THE PATH TO GOOD HEALTH

For the better part of a century, humans have suffered gastrointestinal distress. As time passes, fully processed foods are becoming more and more common in our diet. In addition, our contact with environmental toxins is increasing. Many of these toxins disrupt how our cells communicate, which ultimately disrupts our gastrointestinal health. Awareness of toxins is key to creating a life of wellness, happiness, and joy. We will explore the details as we proceed through this chapter.

Proper TMJ Function Enables the Best Stomach Function

As I alluded to in Chapter One, proper TMJ function is a sign of a balanced pelvis and cranium. These three structures are the keys to a balanced structural system that governs and regulates our autonomic nervous system. As described in Chapter One, the autonomic nervous system is composed of the parasympathetic and sympathetic nervous systems. This chapter explains how the vitality of one's life depends on a healthy autonomic nervous system.

As we have discussed, stomach acid is vital for regulating and sustaining healthy digestion, as is proper TMJ function.

The TMJ is an essential part of the framework in the mouth and throat. Food enters your mouth. After chewing, you swallow it, and it goes down to your esophagus and into your stomach. If the TMJ *subluxates*, or misaligns, this causes a one-sided pull on the neck muscles and the esophagus, which, in turn, can pull the stomach through the diaphragm. In severe cases, this can cause a *hiatal hernia*. This is often the case with infants who have trouble suckling on their mother's breast because of a TMJ issue. The TMJ issue results in gastric reflux.

Whether it is from a hiatal hernia or a less severe TMJ-related problem, the pull on the diaphragm will cause a strain in the stomach lining, resulting in a diminished ability to release sufficient amounts of hydrochloric acid. As described in the next section, stomach acid is a key to attaining the best digestive health.

Proper Stomach Acid Allows for the Best Digestive Health

Stomach acid is a necessity for good digestion. Stomach acid, when stimulated by the parietal cells, causes the stomach environment and its contents to be very acidic, with a pH of roughly 3. This acidity has numerous benefits, including fostering the breakdown of proteins and the neutralization of harmful pathogens that we swallow, such as bacteria, viruses, parasites, and fungi. Finally, stomach acid activates consecutive digestive reflexes, such as the release of digestive enzymes from the pancreas and the gallbladder. It also plays a role in activating the lower bowel to evacuate its contents—resulting in a bowel movement—to prepare for future food contents to enter.

Without proper stomach acid, the body would not be able to digest proteins into amino acids, which are the building blocks to neurotransmitters, immune cells, and hormones. Without these substances to sustain proper blood flow and lymphatic drainage, your organs would be congested, which would ultimately cause a buildup of metabolic waste. Imbalances in the structural system would compound all these problems.

Proper Blood and Lympth Flow Lead to the Best Organ Function

Over my years of offering corrective and supportive care through chiropractic and organ therapies, I have witnessed these treatments enabling the return of normal organ function in patients, as well as better blood flow and lymphatic drainage. I have successfully used these therapies when a patient is suffering from a head cold or even a headache/migraine, which are often a direct result of a congested organ system.

Remember that blood flow can be compromised by a number of inflammatory processes, such as anemia, uncontrolled blood sugar, gastrointestinal issues, infections, and traumas. These increase the body's stress response. These inflammatory processes stress our autonomic nervous system, which can cause blood pressure abnormalities. Blood pressure is never fully corrected until all stomach, intestinal, and colon gases are eliminated.

Carbon dioxide is manufactured in the stomach and reabsorbed in the intestines and colon. Stomach, intestinal, and colon gases are created by abnormalities in digestive chemistry or gut flora.

A body of water that stands still will rapidly become impure. In the same way, blood flow that moves slowly becomes impure, leading to a buildup of toxins and metabolic waste. Proper blood flow and lymphatic drainage are key to having a healthy body and the best organ function. This is why exercise, light or intense, is beneficial to improving blood flow and lymphatic drainage.

This is why health care practitioners often recommend following detoxification programs every few months. These practices are good for those who have already achieved health through lifestyle changes; however, for those who are not healthy, detoxification may create more health problems. A starting place for detoxification for these patients would be abdominal breathing and exercise to increase blood flow; these are good techniques to begin to establish proper blood flow and lymphatic drainage.

A HEALTHY GUT MEANS A STRONGER IMMUNE SYSTEM

Our gastrointestinal tract is responsible for 70 to 80 percent of our immunity.

Many people with chronic health issues have an overworked immune system. The typical protocol is to stimulate the immune system. However, due to the processed foods so many people ingest, the toxic air we breathe, and several other irritants, our immune systems are overworked. This is why turmeric, resveratrol, omega 3 fatty acids, vitamin D, and other antioxidants are of great benefit. They help calm the immune response rather than stimulate our immune cells.

An over-stimulated stress response results in elevated insulin levels, an activated hypothalamic-pituitary-adrenal system, and increased hormone activity. Our gastrointestinal tract is responsible for 70 to 80 percent of our immunity. That immune system depends on a properly working digestive system.

Stomach Acid Is the First Line of Defense

Stomach acid, which has a pH of approximately 3, neutralizes the pathogens that enter the stomach, whether in the form of food, inhaled pollutants, or an ingested antigen. The acid-forming cells of our stomach secrete what is known as mucin, which helps protect the stomach from the acid produced by its own cells. This mucus layer separates the acidic contents from our stomach lining. The breakdown of this mucus layer leads to ulcers.

The breakdown of mucus can be brought on by pathogens, allergies, or stress. The mucus layer is where the beneficial gut microbes live and work synergistically with the immune system. Any breakdown of the mucus barrier decreases the strength of the immune system.

Better Nutrient Absorption Allows for a Stronger Immune System

As mentioned in Chapter One, if the body cannot break down the food into simple molecules, such as amino acids, then the body is unable to make immune cells, neurotransmitters, and hormones, which are the main messengers that regulate our immune system. Among the hundreds of neurotransmitters and hormones in the body, two are especially important to the gut: GABA and serotonin.

These inhibitory neurotransmitters are actually excitatory in the gut. In other words, they decrease the blood flow to the brain while increasing flow to the gut. This may explain why those who have GI problems are sick more often, cannot sleep well, are always tired and irritable, and the list goes on. This brain/gut connection is explained more fully in the next section.

A Healthy Gut Means Better Sleep, Which Improves the Immune System

As noted previously, GABA and serotonin help calm the brain. The brain is a huge mass of connectors with millions, if not billions, of nerves firing to and fro. GABA is a neurotransmitter that helps reduce excess firing between neurons. Glucose, blood sugar, is the principal precursor for the production of GABA, although pyruvate and other amino acids also can act as precursors. The first step is the transamination of an a-ketoglutarate, formed from glucose metabolism in the Krebs cycle.[3] This is why GABA deficiency is the No. 1 complaint of a restless mind, and the best solution for a restless mind is to balance the glucose and insulin response.

Another important neurotransmitter is serotonin. Ninety percent of serotonin is made in the gastrointestinal tract. The other 10 percent of serotonin is made in the brain. The serotonin in our brain helps regulate mood, the sleep/wake cycle, and food intake. These two neurotransmitters are invaluable in managing daily stress and in strengthening immunity while we sleep. Both GABA and serotonin calm down the brain, allowing our brain to enter REM

---

3 Olsen, Richard and Timothy M. DeLorey. "GABA Synthesis, Uptake and Release." *Basic Neurochemistry: Molecular, Cellular, and Medical Aspects.* 6th edition. (Philadelphia: Lippicott-Raven, 1999.)

sleep, which is the preferred method of replenishing and rejuvenating the body and the immune system.

Serotonin is the activator of the stress pathway known as the hypothalamic-pituitary-adrenal axis. Over time, high stress levels, inflammatory processes, and the build-up of toxins will increase the use of this crucial neurotransmitter. This may be the reason so many people are prescribed selective serotonin reuptake inhibitors (SSRIs), which are used as anti-depressants. The need for an SSRI may be an indication of poor gut health.

AN UNHEALTHY GUT AFFECTS MIND AND BODY

The body is a complex system of cells. To function properly, our own cells must work with foreign cells, which we call gut flora. These gut flora consist of good microbes that are very beneficial to the body. They play a major part in nutrient absorption, mood, and even metabolism, as detailed in this section.

Bad Digestion, Bad Microbes, Bad Nutrient Absorption

You now know that a TMJ issue can cause bad digestive chemistry, which can lead to stress, infection, and ultimately a breakdown of the mucus lining of the gastrointestinal system. The thinning of the gastrointestinal lining creates an opening for harmful pathogens and allergies, which will generate inhospitable terrain for the beneficial gut flora.

When given the chance, good bugs become bad bugs. Our gut microbes want to live and thrive. When our pH, stomach acid, and bile salts are altered, the rules change; those beneficial microbes may stop being beneficial.

When the natural checks and balances system is impaired, gut flora that are supposed to stay in the small intestine may travel upward. These bacteria can even travel up into organs, such as the gallbladder, causing formations known as gallstones. This is the cause of gallbladder inflammation. This is also the cause of SIBO or *small intestinal bacterial overgrowth*.

Bacterial diversity involves complex ecosystems, and the topic is beyond the scope of this book, but we can discuss the fundamentals that ensure the gut flora is balanced. A medical professional can test and verify that your stomach acid, pH, and gallbladder function are working well. Probiotics are beneficial to gut health, as are fermented foods. It is worthwhile and extremely beneficial to have both in your daily diet. Foods such as yogurt are low in probiotic quantity. A diverse selection of fermented foods ensures a wide diversity of beneficial microbes for better immunity and absorption of nutrients.

Bad Digestion, Poor Mood

Have you ever met someone who is irritable or easily upset if they miss a meal?

When someone hasn't eaten for a while, neurotransmitters, hormones, and immune cells become scarce because of the lack of amino acids. Often, neurotransmitters are affected most severely, and they can have far-reaching effects on the body.

For example, serotonin, dopamine, and GABA play major roles in our autonomic nervous system related to:

- Digestion
- Sleep
- Energy
- Memory
- Libido
- Learning
- Mood

To expand on this concept, it helps to think of these neurotransmitters as teams. GABA and serotonin are on the *red team* because they are like a stop switch to our central nervous system. Dopamine, norepinephrine, and epinephrine are the *green team* because they are like the gas pedal in a car that goes and goes.

As mentioned in the previous section, inflammation in the gut decreases the ability to make serotonin. Serotonin is a major player on the red team because it dampens our stress response; it also improves nutrient absorption through the blood flow to the gut and allows better quality sleep. GABA, along with serotonin, calms the brain and its stress response. GABA is a key player in settling the mind.

However, dopamine, norepinephrine, and epinephrine are movers and shakers. They are highly excitable because they promote wakefulness, energy, and activity. The nervous system waxes and wanes due to the calming effects of GABA. Through the go-go efforts of our green team, GABA levels can be exhausted, too, along with serotonin. This can create a variety of symptoms, including anxiety, insomnia, and chronic pain patterns.

To summarize, the red team is the body's braking system. It allows us to stop, rest, digest, and repair. The green team is the gas pedal, which promotes energy, libido, and joy for life. If you lose your brakes, this will eventually result in hitting the wall and crashing. At that point, both teams will then need repair. This is a common theme in cases of depression, anxiety, irritability, and many other common mood and behavior cases.

Do you believe mood and behavior can affect how you take care of yourself?

Did you know that mood and behavior can also affect your metabolism?

Bad Gut, Bad Metabolism

> Metabolism is the set of chemical processes that occur through cellular mechanisms to maintain life.

How does gut function relate to metabolism?

To be sure you have a clear picture of how poor digestive chemistry affects nutrient absorption, reread the *Bad Digestion, Bad Microbes, Bad Nutrient Absorption* section.

Next, let's define *metabolism*. Metabolism refers to the set of chemical processes that occur through cellular mechanisms to maintain life. These processes are coordinated by elements of the digestive system, endocrine system, and nervous system.

This section provides more detail about the set of organs that help regulate metabolism.

There are three key elements:

- The gut/brain axis
- The thyroid gland
- The liver

The first of the three key elements is a tag team I will refer to as the gut/brain axis. The gut and the brain are in constant communication through hormones, neurotransmitters, and immune messenger molecules through blood and cerebrospinal fluid (CSF). By maintaining and orchestrating proper digestive chemistry, the body's ability to metabolize increases exponentially. This is why people who eat well, exercise, and take care of their bodies are on the path to a healthy lifestyle.

The second element is the thyroid gland. This gland is the master regulator of metabolism throughout the body. Every cell uses thyroid hormone because every cell must maintain its own metabolism for the system of which it is a part. Stomach inflammation, or *gastritis*, disrupts thyroid hormone production through changes in gastric hormone levels. When the thyroid is functioning poorly or is *hypothyroid*, digestion is hindered due to poor cellular metabolism from inadequate thyroid hormone.

The third regulating element in metabolism is a specific function of the liver: the conversion of thyroid hormone. This process is described below.

The thyroid gland makes two different thyroid hormones, *triiodothyronine* (T3) and *thyroxine* (T4). In a healthy system, the thyroid gland makes approximately 93 percent T4 and 7 percent T3. T3 is the active form, but T4 is not; it must be converted by healthy gut flora and liver processes into T3, which is the form that all cells use to maintain metabolism. Roughly 60 percent of T4 is converted to T3 in the liver.

The conversion of thyroid hormone in the liver is another process that is disrupted by stomach inflammation. You can see why, if the body is full of toxins, if the digestive system is impaired, or if mood and behavior are altered or negative, this will drastically affect metabolism.

> *YES! I highly recommend Drs. Asahara and Weber. They are a caring team of Chiropractors, who have a good grasp of whole person care. They are thorough and cautious with each patient and have done many successful treatments for me and many family and friends.*
>
> F. Long, MD
> Sacramento, CA

CHAPTER THREE

Improve Your Mindset and Improve Your Health

YOU THINK WHAT YOU ARE

The mind is very powerful, more than you might think. In this chapter, we will explore the connection between mind and health. We will discover exactly how negative thoughts and imagery can get in the way of pursuing and achieving optimal health.

Your Body Reflects What You Think and Believe

In the past decade, many books and articles have conveyed the message that what you believe and envision, you can achieve. Books such as Joe Dispenza's *Becoming Supernatural: How Common People Are Doing the Uncommon* (2017), *Think and Grow Rich* (1937) by Napoleon Hill, and *The Biology of Belief: Unleashing the Power of Consciousness, Matter & Miracles* (2005) by Bruce Lipton make this point.

Movies such as Byrne's 2006 film *The Secret* and *What the Bleep Do We Know!?* (2004) are terrific box office hits that explore what the power of the mind can do.

Have you ever uttered words like:

- *I can't do that because I am too tired, stressed, and overworked.*
- *I hurt all over.*
- *I feel worthless.*
- *I can't seem to finish anything I start.*
- *I don't think I will ever get better.*
- *I am ready to give up.*

I have worked with several patients who constantly spoke phrases such as these. It is unfortunate that so many people define themselves by what they don't like or can't do. Those who repeat phrases such as these are limiting themselves. They are *problem-oriented.*

Would you say you are *problem-oriented* or *solution-oriented?*

In other words, when a problem exists, do you become *Captain Obvious* — just restating the problem all the time — or are you the rare person who brings and identifies a solution as well as the problem?

It is important to understand that you may be impeding your health through your mindset. You can't achieve an increased level of wellness if you maintain a problem-oriented mindset.

> *The definition of insanity is doing the same thing over and over again and expecting different results.*
>
> ~ widely attributed to Albert Einstein

Everything is energy, including words and thoughts. Simply opening the mind's thought process to a different belief changes the energy in the body, enabling new habits to form.

If you are reading this book, you are probably looking for a way to improve your health. I would bet that you have tried to change your habits. Perhaps you began an exercise routine, you tried to create better sleep habits, or you tried to relieve your stress in some way, shape, or form. This probably made you feel better for a time.

My questions for you are these:

- Why didn't you stay with it?
- Was it too hard?
- Were you not seeing the results you intended to achieve?

Consider whether you envisioned yourself getting better, or whether you foresaw yourself reverting to your old habits even before you started. This is an example of *intending* to change, but perhaps not *believing* you could change. Intention is not enough; the belief is necessary for your body to get there.

Tired of Being Tired

As I discussed in the last chapter, high stress levels activate the release of high cortisol levels from the neuroadrenal cortex. A large amount of cortisol released in the blood causes insulin receptor sites to be defective, which develops into insulin receptor site insensitivity, otherwise known as *insulin resistance,* which is the start of diabetes mellitus type 2.

In times of insulin resistance, the body's insulin receptor sites do not respond appropriately to insulin; therefore, the pancreas releases more insulin to push glucose into the cells.

This results in a negative shift in the entire metabolic process, causing:

- Higher levels of insulin

- A massive shift in electrolytes, contributing to muscle cramps and dehydration

- Faulty detoxification mechanisms

- Fat deposition around organs and muscles, causing weight gain and organ congestion

- Leptin resistance, decreasing the feeling of fullness after a meal

After a time, when cortisol levels have been exhausted, leading to adrenal fatigue or adrenal exhaustion, the exhaustion phase will cause a monstrous negative effect on the body and its ability to stabilize glucose levels. Remember, cortisol is responsible for raising blood glucose levels in times of fasting or long absences of meals. Adrenal exhaustion diminishes the body's ability to stabilize glucose levels. Two phenomena — *hypoglycemia* and *hyperglycemia*--set up the body for a metabolic disaster.

Hypoglycemia, or low glucose, leads to adrenal exhaustion, and hyperglycemia, or high glucose, leads to high cortisol levels, ultimately causing hormone changes in the gastrointestinal tract, the brain, and all systems dealing with metabolism. With this hormone change also comes a shift in neurotransmitters and immune cells. This causes the main governing system of the body to be impaired.

To present this another way, picture yourself finishing your last year of college. You are expecting your first child within the next month or two. Passing three of your classes weighs heavily on your getting the grade point average that you need to qualify for the best positions in your field of study. With this stress, your eating habits begin to suffer. Sandwiches and chocolates become your coping mechanisms. You notice your loose-fitting jeans become your tight-fitting jeans. You also begin to notice that your memory is not as sharp as it was even a month ago. You are easily irritated. No matter how much sleep you get, you are still tired.

What would you do in a scenario like this?

You might want to lose weight, so you might start exercising and working out by lifting weights. Working out will burn calories; however, stress decreases thermic efficiency, which is your body's ability to burn calories and metabolize stored fat. In addition, worrying about weight gain is a stressor, and therefore sends your body into a greater stress response—one result is increased fat deposits or weight gain.

Many people use anxiety and stress to motivate themselves to lose weight. This will ultimately cause an overwhelming feeling of exhaustion, which results in being tired of being tired. We must train our bodies as well as our minds to reach a healthier level.

Your Body Is an Amazing Beautiful Machine—Don't Waste It

> *You can give a person knowledge, but you can't*
> *make them think. Some people want to remain*
> *fools, only because the truth requires change.*
> ~ Tony A. Gaskins, Jr.

After reading this book, you will begin to understand what great power for healing your body holds. As a doctor, I cannot heal your body; only you have that power.

Like all games, including the game of life, coaches and mentors can help us improve how we play the game. In this game of life that we all play, how we go about our health is up to us. Doctors like myself have dedicated our lives to help you regain yours. Therefore, you and I, the doctor, must work as a team to achieve the best possible outcome. The best quality of life that we can hope for is to live a disease-free life and, eventually, die a peaceful death.

Think about these questions:

- If you cut yourself, is it the bandage that heals you?
- Is it the doctor that heals you?
- Is it the medicine that heals you?

The answer to these questions is no.

All those elements help the body heal, but think about this: *If you were dead, would any of those factors help heal you?*

The answer, of course, is no.

> *The state of your individual health is spiritually/ vibrationally induced, chemically/electrically driven, and biologically carried out.*
>
> ~ "Blood and Consciousness"
> Biomedix.com (October 19, 2000)

The body is made up of ten systems, according to the Western medical model. Alternative forms of healing recognize there is also a mental/emotional aspect to health, and, in addition, there is a spiritual element to health. Our biomechanical system, our mental/ emotional health, and our spiritual health make us the beautiful creatures we are.

The body has a greater power than you can ever imagine. You create conscious thought. Your brain then programs this thought through a cellular system, which results in the body carrying out the order. This is why it is important that your mindset be prepared before you start a health program; this mindset will help you achieve your desired results and keep them.

These topics are explored in greater depth in a later chapter.

LONG-TERM STRESS LEADS TO POOR HEALTH

By the time we reach the age of seven, our nervous system has become our adult nervous system. Every distortion pattern that we attain as a child, we are living with as an adult. Many patients we see in our office have a long-term stress issue that needs to be dealt with in order to make any type of optimal health changes to their body. This section explores those aspects.

Long-Term Stress Decreases Communication Between Systems

In a previous section, I introduced the nervous system, the hormonal system, and the immune system as our governing systems; they are your body's communication network. In this section, I want to explore how long-term stress weighs heavily on this governing system. I will term this three-tiered communication system the neuro-endocrine-immune system.

You may remember that our nervous system uses neurotransmitters to relay what it wants and what it needs to other systems. The endocrine system, or our hormonal system, communicates through a vast array of hormones numbering in the several hundreds. The last governing system is our immune system, which communicates through immune cells, such as cytokines, chemokines, and adipokines.

As I stated in an earlier chapter, 80 percent of our immune system is in our gastrointestinal tract. Long-term stress has a detrimental effect on the immune system. It decreases the expression of insulin on receptor sites. It increases the expression of inflammatory cytokines such as interleukin-6. It decreases production of interleukin-12 and interleukin gamma, which are necessary for fighting cellular infections.

Long-term stress also increases activation of the stress response, the hypothalamic-pituitary-adrenal (HPA) axis.

This causes:

- Suppressed luteinizing hormone in males, which dampens testosterone production
- Suppressed luteinizing hormone in females, which decreases progesterone levels
- Depleted mineral supplies
- Suppressed white blood cells
- Elevated C-reactive proteins
- Disrupted mitochondrial energy production

- Decreased iron, hemoglobin, and other complete blood count lab values
- Disrupted production of dopamine, norepinephrine, and epinephrine, which are our energy neurotransmitters
- Altered serotonin levels in the brain
- An imbalanced autonomic nervous system
- Altered use of essential fatty acids
- Disrupted gut healing and digestive enzyme function

This is a condensed list of what long-term stress does to your body. If this does not scare you, I encourage you to research more. Our body can handle long-term stress when all systems work as they should. However, the body is only as strong as the weakest link; it is only as strong as the weakest system.

A great analogy to illustrate this point is the check engine light in your car.

Does your car still run with the check engine light on?

Absolutely — but *for how long* is the question. Often, it takes a mechanical diagnostician to determine why the check engine light is on. The same goes for our bodies. It takes a well-educated diagnostician to understand the depths of your anatomy and physiology.

Your body, like a car, has safeguards that function when something is not running optimally. This means that when something is wrong, the body may still work, but there will be warning signs that show you that there is a problem. When your car check engine light is on, you can go to your neighborhood automotive shop to get it turned off, but this doesn't fix the problem. In the same way, you can ignore warning signs in your body, but this won't solve your health problems.

Long-Term Stress Is a Vicious Cycle

In the previous section, I listed for you several items that are altered with long-term stress. That list is not complete by any means, but I hope it paints a picture that clearly shows that stress is a vicious cycle.

When one area of your body falls short, another part picks up the slack until it reaches its breaking point, then another part will try to pick up the slack, and so on. Reducing stressors of all kinds—biomechanical, biochemical, mental, emotional—will help reduce the impact of the vicious cycle of long-term stress. It is on you, the master of your own body, to begin turning big stressors into minute obstacles so your body can heal and become strong.

How can you accomplish such a monumental task?

Simple. The same way you eat an elephant — one bite at a time.

> *A journey of a thousand miles begins with a single step.*
>
> ~ Lao Tzu

To begin, at this very moment, you can start by changing your thoughts about yourself. Stress in this life is inevitable. The two items that you have control over are your thoughts and actions.

Next, address the health of your biomechanical system. Set up an appointment with your chiropractor or your osteopath. According to my knowledge, in the United States, these are the only two professionals allowed to adjust the muscular system — chiropractors and osteopaths. There is no good way to find a good adjuster. The same method is used to find a contractor or plumber — try. No two doctors are the same, which is why the doctor and you should agree on the course of therapy. Second and even third opinions may be necessary.

Once you have made sure your biomechanical system has been finely tuned, now focus on your internal biochemistry. Lab analysis is always a safe way to go. It is better to test rather than guess.

It's also important to find a practitioner who understands lab results and treatments. Many patients come to me after attempting to improve their health by taking supplements, basing their selections solely on what was promoted as being the best in the market. After spending hundreds of dollars — if not thousands — they have often seen no improvement at all in lab values.

In our office, we have a checklist of body chemistry items to look at and address as needed.

Common items that require assessment are:

- Inflammation
- Anemia
- Glucose
- Adrenal function
- Metabolic regulators: thyroid, liver detox
- Digestive chemistry

A majority of people with a long-term health issue usually also have anemia or a blood sugar imbalance, so these are two areas we will assess first. Anemia reduces the oxygen-carrying capacity of the blood. Oxygen is a necessary component of life. If the body does not have sufficient amounts of oxygen, it cannot support the biochemical reactions and normal daily activities of the body.

Second on the list is glucose. This test helps us assess the stress response that is governed by the patient's adrenal glands. If glucose levels are abnormal, then cellular metabolism will be compromised, which adds more stress to our neuro-endocrine-immune system. Our bodies release cortisol in response to stress.

A third priority is the patient's metabolizing regulators, which include liver detoxification pathways, thyroid metabolism, and digestion. It is crucial that your body has the capability to eliminate toxins that enter your body by ingestion, through the skin, or in the air we breathe. It is equally important that thyroid hormone be properly regulated since it is the gas pedal of our body. When the thyroid gland makes more thyroid hormone, your metabolic rate increases. When it slows down, so does the production of thyroid hormone.

The next part to focus on is digestion. If your body cannot digest and absorb the necessary nutrients, then your body is breaking down from the inside out. This is also known as malnutrition.

The last section on our body chemistry priority checklist is the immune system. Lab markers show whether your immune system needs repair. Patients dealing with an autoimmune condition or chronic health issue often need to calm down the immune system and not stimulate it. Other times, the immune system may need to be stimulated. It is only by running lab tests that we truly know what the body's immune system is facing. Otherwise, a seasoned clinician may know based on presentation, but they will be more accurate after running the tests.

Test! Don't guess! You will save money in the long run.

By going through this checklist, we can be sure that your body is making the necessary strides to regain its vitality and break the vicious cycle of stress.

Decreasing Stress Improves Metabolism

As we begin to build up your health profile, we explore other players that will improve cellular metabolism.

The major players I have found in clinical practice include:

- Exercise
- Avoidance of stress stimulators
- Relaxation techniques

These three factors, when applied to your daily life, will greatly improve mental clarity, energy levels, and your overall health.

First, I want to discuss *exercise*. I strongly recommend every individual have at least two different types of exercise routines. For example, weight lifting and cardio are a good combination, while squats and pushups, both anaerobic exercises, would not work well together. Cycling and running would be too similar as well.

For improving cellular metabolism, you should choose one activity that increases your heart rate — without straining — while still strengthening your body at a mild heart rate or moderate blood pressure. Your aerobic activity should increase your heart rate to approximately 60 percent of your maximum heart rate.

You can easily calculate your maximum heart rate. Subtract your age from 220, and this equals your maximum heart rate. For instance, if you are 30 years old, your maximum heart rate is 190 beats per minute. Since we've said your aerobic activity should increase your heart rate to 60 percent of your maximum heart rate, in this example, you should be aiming for 60 percent of 190, which is 114 beats per minute.

This moderate level of exercise will reduce your cortisol levels compared to any level of exercise that raises your heartrate above 70 percent, which raises cortisol levels. This is one of the items we teach our patients who enter this program.

The second aspect to improving metabolism is *avoiding stress stimulators* such as:

- Concentrated sugars
- Caffeine—including decaffeinated coffee, which still has some caffeine
- Nicotine
- Alcohol
- Allergen foods—because histamine is a stress stimulant
- Partially hydrogenated foods—which block the production of steroid hormones
- Artificial sweeteners
- Overtraining
- Inadequate sleep

All these topics increase stress while weakening the neuro-endocrine-immune system.

Relaxation techniques are supporters of good metabolism. You might try yoga, deep-breathing exercises, meditation, or tai chi. All these techniques help to reduce stress levels in the body. These are particularly useful for individuals with a chronic injury or disability, allowing improved mental relaxation and clarity. As these techniques are engaged properly, they improve blood flow and lymph, provide better oxygenation to tissues, and strengthen neural receptors in the brain, which helps balance the autonomic nervous system.

LIVE WELL AND BE HAPPY

By this point in the book, I hope you have begun to see the complexity of the body, and are aware of the obstacles that your body faces, but also see that there is a light at the end of the tunnel. You have the power to improve your health. You can build a stronger way of life. As we begin to build an optimized wellness plan for you, keep these factors in mind.

Movement Is a Key to Good Health

Our bodies were designed to move. One of the biggest problems in today's society is a lack of movement. We live an increasingly sedentary lifestyle. In total, Americans are sitting an average of thirteen hours a day and sleeping an average of eight hours a night, resulting in a sedentary lifestyle twenty-one hours per day. While Americans know about the importance of exercise, only 31 percent go to the gym, and 56 percent devote less than ten dollars a month to staying active.[4]

The scientific community has coined the term *sitting disease*, referring to a metabolic syndrome that is due to the ill effects of an overly sedentary lifestyle. A 2013 survey from Ergotron found that of the vast majority of people surveyed, approximately 93 percent didn't know what sitting disease was, but 74 percent believed that sitting too much could lead to an early death.[5]

As I mentioned in Chapter One, the human body relies on a perfectly working mechanical system. The best way to support the mechanical system is to make sure it can move. Arthritis and stiff joints are the fastest ways to reduce movement in any individual. In every joint lives a specific type of cell called a *chondrocyte*. These cells are special because of their ability to build cartilage.

Can you guess what the easiest way is to stimulate chondrocytes to build cartilage?

---

4 "New Survey: To Sit or Stand? Almost 70% of Full Time American Workers Hate Sitting but They do it all Day Every Day." *Ciston: PR Newswire.* 17 July 2013. prnewswire.com/news-releases/new-survey-to-sit-or-stand-almost-70-of-full-time-american-workers-hate-sitting-but-they-do-it-all-day-every-day-215804771.html
5 Ergotron JustStand Survey & Index Report. 07/15/2013. juststand.org/wp-content/uploads/2017/05/SurveyIndexReport.pdf.

If you guessed *movement,* you are right. Every individual living with an arthritic joint should slowly begin to move, which will activate the making of cartilage or discs between joints. Begin slowly and gradually increase according to your own abilities. If needed, consult your doctor or another health care provider.

Proper Digestion, Proper Nutrition, Better Sleep

In Chapter Two, we discussed the importance of digestive chemistry and the making of neurotransmitters, specifically GABA and serotonin. As we have already learned, the making of stomach acid allows the breakdown of proteins to begin. This, in turn, activates the release of digestive enzymes from the pancreas so the proteins can continue to break down into amino acids.

Accordingly, it is of great importance to know which factors cause a lack of stomach acid production. The failure of digestive chemistry is the domino that begins the cascade that knocks over so many digestive processes.

Items that may impair stomach acid production include the following:

- A psoas/diaphragm contraction
- Eating foods that are too cold or drinking ice water before or with a meal
- Taking antacids fairly regularly
- B-vitamin deficiencies
- Eating in between meals
- Eating a diet too high in protein
- Any irritation of the stomach lining
- Stress

A psoas/diaphragm contraction may cause a hiatal hernia, causing muscle distortion throughout the body. Eating between meals or eating a diet too high in protein will eventually exhaust the cells in the stomach that make hydrochloric acid.

Stress increases the stress response, which activates the sympathetic nervous system. This, in turn, shuts off digestive processes. It can be helpful for some people to avoid watching active movies while they eat. Any irritation of the stomach lining will decrease the production of mucus that enables gut flora bacteria to flourish without boundaries.

If you make an effort to correct or avoid these items, your digestion will be far more efficient. The proper stomach acid level allows the body to activate the necessary digesting sequence that leads to greater nutrient absorption. As good nutrients are absorbed, this results in better detoxification mechanisms, better healing capabilities, and more importantly, better sleep. Also, remember that eating according to the seasons helps allow for better nutrient absorption throughout the year, and this is another key to long-term health.

Good Digestive Chemistry Allows for Happier Cells

Long-term stressors often impede the use of serotonin and dopamine in the brain's frontal cortex. This often leads to a decreased number of neurons firing, causing signs and symptoms of depression.

Do you believe our society uses too many anti-depressants?

According to a 2018 analysis of federal data by *The New York Times,* some 15.5 million people have been taking medications for at least five years. The results have almost doubled since 2010 and more than tripled since 2000. Nearly 25 million adults have been on anti-depressants for at least two years, a 60 percent increase since 2010.[6]

---

6 Carvey, Benedict and Robert Gebeloff. "Many People Taking Antidepressants Discover They Cannot Quit." *The New York Times.* April 7, 2018. nytimes.com/2018/04/07/health/antidepressants-withdrawal-prozac-cymbalta.html

Depression has been studied extensively by neurologists in several fields. They have determined one of the primary contributing factors in depression is diminished firing of the frontal lobe of the brain. The frontal lobe makes up the front third of the brain. This part of the brain is responsible for motor function and planning.

The frontal lobe also determines important qualities like:

- Judgment
- Determination
- Concentration
- Curiosity
- Motivation
- Mental flexibility
- Personality
- Planning
- Organization
- Sequencing of working memory

Serotonin and dopamine have a great influence on neurons in the frontal lobe. Neurons associated with serotonin are important for pain modulation and the production of melatonin. Imbalances in these neurons may lead to insomnia, altered heat regulation, and behavioral changes as the seasons change throughout the year, including changes in sexual activity. Neurons associated with dopamine receptors are used to activate our muscular system, and to evoke emotional responses such as a sense of reward and pleasure, along with regulating our personality traits.

You may be wondering: *Okay, how does this all play into digestion and happier cells?*

Foods like snapper, chicken breast, and liver are high in an amino acid called *tryptophan,* which is a precursor to making serotonin in the gut as well as in the brain. Dopamine is also made from an amino acid, phenylalanine, which is dependent on proper digestive chemistry. If your body cannot break down your food into amino acids, then your frontal lobe, as well as the rest of your body, will be lacking essential amino acids that make powerful neurotransmitters like serotonin and dopamine. A healthy digestive tract leads to a happy brain, along with a happy body.

The body is a complex system. Often, people would prefer to determine that it's just one thing that causes their ailment. But the fact of the matter is it is never just one thing. It is everything at once. So be aware of everything that is happening to you so you can improve your mind as well as your body.

It's never just one thing; it is everything at once.

~ Morihei Ueshiba, O' Sensei
Founder of Akido

I visited Quantum Chiropractic after suffering with leg soreness, shortness of breath, and trouble falling asleep (insomnia) for three years. My leg soreness and ability to fall asleep improved in four months and are now resolved after working with Dr. Jim and Dr. Pauline on both Chiropractic care and nutrition. They were the only ones that have helped — I visited four other doctors: cardiologist, pulmonary, massage specialist, and chiropractor.

My son has never liked eating. At the age of six he is in the fourteenth percentile in height and tenth percentile in weight on his growth chart. It was such a struggle; I would have to distract him with an iPad and spoon feed him to get him to eat. Since we have been working with Dr. Pauline, he has been eating more without assistance. The biggest improvement that has been noticed by family, teachers, and friends has been his temperament.

Thank you so much, Dr. Jim and Dr. Pauline,
for helping me and my family!

A. Liston
Sacramento, CA

CHAPTER FOUR

Long-Term Wellness Takes Discipline

LIKE MARTIAL ARTS, GOOD HEALTH REQUIRES DISCIPLINE

I have been practicing martial arts for most of my life, and it's been amazing to see the vast differences, but more importantly, the similarities of not only the structure but the discipline, and constant practice to make sure every effort you do is for the best of the movement, for the best of protecting your life.

Of course, many of us think martial arts are just for defense. But in the same mindset of your health, offense is the best defense. Being proactive about your health will be the best thing you can do to protect your health for the long haul.

Structure Is the Key to Good Movement

Every good martial artist knows that solid structure and proper form are the keys to performing any particular movement. The musculoskeletal system of martial artists, like that of other athletes, is often finely tuned because of a highly complex network of cellular receptor sites that make up the *proprioceptor* system.

Proprioception literally means *sense of self.* A group of sensor modalities in the proprioceptor system allows us to know the positions of our limbs in space. It senses our movements and enacts protective forces automatically. Our proprioceptor system is like a home security system, which scatters alarm sensors all over our body.

Remember that we have 206 bones in our body, and at every bone-to-bone contact is a joint. If you do the math, we have a lot of joints. Each of them has an associated proprioceptor system.

For example, consider the *acetabulum* or hip joint. Allow me to draw out a picture of this particular joint. In each of our hips, there are approximately 156 proprioceptors, which include a total of 312 proprioceptors from both hips that inform the brain where it is in time and space in relationship to everything around it. This information informs the brain of blood flow, gas pressure in the blood vessels, tissue integrity, and so much more.

If the hip becomes problematic—if it subluxates, for instance—this then creates a whole host of complicating factors. The hip joint is the closest joint to the trunk. When this joint becomes problematic, everything down the line, including the knee, ankle, and foot, can also become problematic. To add further complication, the muscles that attach to the hip joint are many of our core muscles, which are major players in back spasms and other forms of low back pain.

With two hip joints that are balanced, the eyes rest easily on the horizon. When one hip joint is problematic, then the eyes become unleveled, leading to balance issues, TMJ dysfunction, upper neck pains, abnormal shoulder mobility, and the list goes on. When a joint is out of balance, the deterioration of nerve endings begins, which causes a cascade of disrupted proprioceptors along a kinetic chain.

It is impossible for the nervous system or circulatory system to function normally with an imbalanced kinetic chain. The health of these proprioceptors is vital for joint maintenance for the neuro-endocrine-immune system that we discussed previously.

Exercise, chiropractic, stretching, yoga, tai chi, massage, acupuncture, and other therapies may help in the maintenance and healing of these specialized nerve cells called proprioceptors. The chiropractic adjustment, however, is the best healing modality for these specialized receptors because, unlike most other healing modalities, the adjustment puts the joint back in close proximity.

Good Movement Is the Best Defense

Exercise is undoubtedly good for everyone, but many people don't understand why this is so, or what kind of exercise is most beneficial. Often, most people just assume running and lifting weights is the best for all of us.

Consider these questions:

- What does exercise do to our bodies that allows us to function better?
- What does exercise do for our immune cells?
- Will exercise harm us?

As I discussed in the last section, our bodies were made to move. For simplicity's sake, let's break exercise down into three intensity categories: light, moderate, and high. The level of intensity should be calculated based on your maximum heart rate, which, as we've already reviewed, can be estimated by subtracting your age from 220.

Doing low-intensity exercise, your heart rate should reach 40–50 percent of the maximum heart rate. You should reach 50–70 percent of your maximum heart rate during moderate-intensity exercise, and at high intensity, 70–85 percent of your maximum heart rate.

For instance, for a forty-year-old, maximum heart rate is 180 beats per minute. A low- intensity workout should reach about 85 beats per minute, 108 beats per minute for moderate intensity, and 135 beats per minute for a high-intensity workout.

Moderate-intensity exercise is best for most individuals to experience a beneficial physiological response. Moderate-intensity exercise can include weight training, endurance exercises like jogging and cycling, or even swimming. Ideally, we want you to do 150 minutes of moderate activity every week to get the best results.

An article from the Department of Infectious Diseases in Copenhagen evaluated immune cells during and after exercise. The concentration of white blood cells, which are our soldiers facing disease on the front line, increased during exercise. Neutrophils, which are the immune cells that go to infection sites to devour infectious pathogens, increased fourfold after exercising. Natural killer cells, which are white blood cells that play a major role in immunity against tumors and viruses, doubled during exercise activity and returned to normal two hours after physical activity had stopped. Monocytes, which are our immune system's garbage trucks, cleaning up the waste and debris during times of infectious disease, increased two to three times following exercise.[7]

What does all this mean?

Moderate levels of exercise boost immunity.

In addition, moderate levels of exercise have been shown to lower blood pressure, improve cholesterol levels, prevent bone loss, improve energy levels, and maintain mental well-being. If you are sick or feeling ill, exercise may be your best defense. Perhaps a day or two of moderate exercise activity will help you improve quicker than a round of antibiotics. All in all, regular exercise activity is a good way to optimize your health.

---

7 Pedersen, B.K. "Influence of physical activity on the cellular immune system: mechanisms of action." *PubMed: US National Library of Medicine.* ncbi.nlm.nih.gov/pubmed/1894394

Focus on the *Now* so You Can Live Tomorrow

One day at aikido practice, my friend and I were practicing a weapons kata, or form. As we were practicing the kata for about the third time, my sensei yelled, "Chigao!"

In Japanese, this means *wrong*.

My classmate and I looked at each other, puzzled because we had not changed our moves since we had started. My sensei explained. It wasn't that the sequence of movements was wrong; it was our *focus* that needed improvement.

We must focus on every moment as if it could be our last. This way you can live until the next one. Make sure that every movement puts us in a good position before you take the next move. This simple form echoed not only in my training as a student of martial arts, but as a doctor and as a husband.

Take a moment to consider your focus.

How well do you focus on *the now?*

Do you have a to-do list that is a mile long and is growing by the second?

Do you take care of yourself first before taking care of everyone else?

If you have a big heart, more than likely, you put yourself last. I did this same thing growing up, and into adulthood, until halfway through my chiropractic college. At that time, I found my fasting glucose elevated, which made me pre-diabetic — also known as insulin-resistant. This is when I took an in-depth look at my life and had to ask some hard questions:

How I was going to help anyone if I didn't help myself?

What good is a doctor or teacher of medicine that cannot think or help others find a solution to their health problems?

How could I be a good doctor if I couldn't think, recall information, or even practice what I was preaching to my patients?

The simple answer to each of these questions was *I couldn't.*

If you are a planner, that is a great trait. But please do not forget about the present. If I had a quarter for every time I heard a patient say: *I will get to that, I will start that as soon as I get this done,* or *when I get back from vacation,* I would have a lot of quarters. We all tend to invent excuses that push off what needs to start today.

You are alive, right this second. In case you are unsure, check your pulse and spend a moment focusing on your breathing. You are alive, so you can fight. You can start to build a healthier life for yourself, right now.

By reading this book, you are taking action to prevent ill health. You are choosing to be proactive in building a long and healthy life for yourself. Every activity you endure, every food particle you ingest, every thought you think will help or hinder your health. By focusing on a better quality of health now, you will ensure that you will have a better life to live tomorrow.

Facts and information about your health should ideally make sense to you. Health and well-being should make sense, which is why being healthy is simple. The most difficult aspect is avoiding the pitfalls and landmines society has put forth to all of us.

SLOW AND STEADY WINS THE RACE

Many times, we want very fast results, and we are willing to do whatever is necessary to get those fast results.

However, when you build a house too fast, what happens to the house?

It crumbles. It is not good quality. Take the time to do it right the first time. That way, you don't have to keep chasing your tail and keep fixing what you didn't get right the first time.

It Takes Time to Heal

It takes time to build a situation of ill health in your body, and it will take even longer to heal.

Many of us have fallen, lifted, or bumped into something that causes us pain. It is the obscure pain that causes us to scratch our heads. I often have patients telling me: *Hey, Doc. I woke up this morning, and I couldn't turn my head. I don't know what I did.*

This scenario is one that you may have experienced yourself, or perhaps have heard someone else complain about. The likelihood that this individual fell or sustained some kind of injury while sleeping is very unlikely.

So, what causes this kind of stiff neck?

Keeping the differential diagnosis short, we can assume it was something the patient did prior to waking up that morning. The point of the story is not to diagnose him, but to expand our awareness past the belief that only physical trauma can cause muscle tension.

In previous chapters, I have explained how our organ systems, when stressed, may cause muscle spasms to occur. This is often the case for individuals like the one I am describing here at the beginning of this section.

The majority of those who can pinpoint their pain to an area less than a quarter often turn out to have a musculoskeletal problem that, when therapy is done correctly, will improve very quickly — in days if not hours.

In contrast, those individuals who describe their pain pattern as covering an area larger than the size of their palm are often found to be suffering from a nutritional or organ imbalance. This causes muscle tightness in specific areas of the body.

For example, when a person with high or low blood sugar is describing their pain areas, you may hear them describe:

- Inside knee pain
- Between the shoulder blades pain
- Abdominal pain
- Pain under the left side of the rib cage
- Pain on the left side of the neck
- Headaches on both sides above the ears

Why do they feel pain in so many places?

Nutritionally deprived patients usually hurt all over because their health issues have been occurring for a while, and this has begun to impact multiple organ systems. These are patients who often are constantly changing their eating habits, are taking mountains of supplements, and are often trying other remedies as well. Commonly, these individuals are suffering from a chronically inflamed gut system with a very low diversity in gut microbiome. They have lost their ability to digest and absorb nutrients, leading to a depletion of amino acids and other nutrients that normally help protect and restore their health. This, of course, doesn't occur overnight; it takes time to break down our organ systems.

The good news is, as long as you are conscious, you can still fight. When mentored correctly, you can gain a lot of ground and rebuild your health.

Small Improvements Every Day Will Build Good Health

Let's look at some small strategies you can use to improve your health. The most practical improvement you can make for your health is to reduce inflammation in every possible way. To hammer this point home, think about how hard it would be to rebuild a house when it is still on fire. Put out that fire—reduce inflammation—and you will definitely see an improvement in your health.

As you have read, the gastrointestinal system is critical in supporting your health. Once you lose your gut health, you are at a far greater risk for pains, cardiovascular disease, dementia, weight gain, skin issues—and the list goes on for about ten more pages.

Cysteine, glutathione, turmeric, resveratrol, and omega-3s are all items that will assist your efforts to reduce inflammation. In your daily regimen, you can support your gut mucosal health through supplementation with items like L-glutamine, aloe vera, deglycerized licorice, and rhubarb officinale, to name a few.

You may be wondering about probiotics. Probiotics are important, but research has shown that fermented foods are more beneficial in comparison. Most probiotics sold over the counter are single strains of bacteria, while fermented foods contain multiple strains that encourage a diverse microbiome. The greater the diversity of your gut microflora, the better your gut integrity, which protects you against issues like leaky gut.

Exercising at a moderate intensity improves blood flow and lymph flow throughout the body. Exercise also stimulates the frontal lobe of the brain, which helps eliminate signs and symptoms of depression, as well as poor thinking habits.

It is important to highlight that stress is a No. 1 killer these days. There are multiple ways to handle stress, from camping to comedy movies to exercise, and so much more. One stress-relieving method we believe works extremely well is meditation. You can research to find experts on meditation, from whom you can learn more about advanced techniques. I will highlight a very simple technique here.

Find a comfortable seat, preferably one where you can sit up straight with your feet on the ground. Take a deep breath, inhaling through your nose and exhaling through your mouth. Start by focusing on your feet. As you breathe, focus on relaxing the muscles in your feet. Allow the tension to fade with each exhalation. After your feet relax, move up to your calves. Repeat the same breathing process.

With every exhalation, allow the muscle tension to leave with your breath. Continue to release all the muscles throughout your body with each exhalation. Move your focus up to your thighs, then to your pelvis, all the way to your head. Continue to concentrate on your breath; your breath is extremely powerful when used correctly. Allow your thoughts to fade with every exhalation. This simple meditation will help you release unknown tension that has been long stored in your body.

These four simple remedies — repair gut health, exercise, meditate, and reduce inflammation through dietary supplements — can make a dramatic impact to your health if you incorporate them into your daily routine.

Structural Care Supports Long-Term Function

Does an efficiently functioning system build a stronger body structure, or does a strong structure foster a better functioning?

There has always been lively argument among practitioners about this subject. Allow me to delve into some of these topics, and you can decide.

On one side, we have to realize that a balanced structural system allows for even muscle contraction, which allows for ideal blood flow and lymphatic drainage. As muscles become unbalanced due to biomechanical stressors like bending and lifting, blood flow is then reduced, and structures like nerves and muscles become irritable, resulting in spasms and pain. These chronic spasms lead to a weakened structural system, which impairs function overall.

On the flip side, we have to look at optimal function to support a balanced structure. The body is held together through fascia trains. Fascia trains are multiple muscle groups, connected by connective tissue, that work as a solitary unit. This fascia unit is highly sensitive to physiological imbalances, like anemias, blood sugar imbalances, infections, and more. When these highly complex fascia trains are shortened due to a nutritional imbalance, this impacts our structural stability. Inflammation also impacts stability by breaking down structural proteins inside our ligaments, which lowers the quality of our ligament strength. This is why the slightest trauma may result in severe instability in some individuals.

This brings us back full circle.

As ligaments are weakened due to long-term structural imbalances, muscles must take on the responsibility of joint stability, resulting in constant muscle tension or tightness. This constant state of contraction often results in one's body feeling fatigued or run-down.

So, which side of the argument do you find yourself on after reading this section?

> *No one area of the body can be separated from the whole.*
>
> ~ Dr. Major Bertnand DeJarnette
> Founder of SORSI

The body is a complex system that relies on every cell to function optimally for long-term use.

KNOWING YOUR BODY IS THE WAY TO GOOD HEALTH

One of the best things a doctor can do for his patients is to help them understand what their body is telling them. Communication is the key to knowing what good health is and what it's not. In this section, we are going to talk about three different facets of communication our bodies deal with. Let us begin.

Understand What Your Body Is Trying to Tell You

When I was a teenager, my uncle Dale told me that if I wanted to know how to fix something, I needed to understand how it worked. When I got into chiropractic school, it was my goal to learn as much as I could. One lesson taught by several of my teachers was the importance of listening to what the body was trying to tell us. I call this *following the indicators*. Pain, of course, is an indicator understood by most of us. Pain is effective in letting you know that something is wrong, but there is something better, although it is much more subtle. It is muscle tightness.

Muscle tightness is an *indicator*. Indicators are stress points in or around joints and muscles. A trigger point in a muscle is an example of an indicator.

The trigger point in a muscle belly is an indication that there is muscle distortion present. Whether it is early- or late-stage, muscle distortion will lead to further health complications. Muscle tightness or muscle tension is the precursor before pain. This is why muscle tightness or tension is a better indicator than pain. Do not ignore muscle tightness or trigger points. They are a form of communication spoken by your body, informing you of ills that are to come.

Your Body Knows What It Wants, Not What It Craves

Continuing with the theme of communication in this section, I want to discuss the common misconceptions surrounding cravings. Many believe that if you crave a food, it must contain a nutrient that is needed by your body. This is not necessarily true; in fact, a craving might indicate exactly the opposite situation.

There are multiple complex physiological pathways associated with cravings. There is an area of the brain called the *hypothalamus,* which is associated with food, emotions, and mood. This region of the brain regulates feelings for both hunger and anxiety centers in the brain.

The hypothalamus is loaded with receptors for both neurotransmitters and hormones that influence eating behaviors. Hormones that regulate your food intake include leptin, insulin, cholecystokinin, and ghrelin. All of them are made in the gut and are used to stimulate areas of the brain that impact our wants and needs. These hormones control fat usage and storage as well. These are additional reasons why a healthy gut is the best way to optimize your health.

The gut hormones are signaled by multiple systems; the big players are your nervous system, immune system, hormones, and microbiome. These systems are influenced by your stress pathways, as well as the quality and quantity of available nutrients. If your body's nutrient concentration is low, then hormone signaling will increase, and the intensity of your hunger will dramatically increase, producing a craving. The signal goes to your brain, specifically your hypothalamus, and puts you in the mood for your favorite dish.

The definition of a craving is a powerful desire for something.

Have you ever noticed that we rarely crave steak, salad, or vegetables?

To put it simply, we generally don't crave what we think of as *real* food. We are much more likely to crave things like chocolate, or salty or sugary snacks. Sugar, specifically, is an example of a powerful stimulator of excitatory neurons that produce strong urges and desires. These excitatory neurons are your *go-go* neurons within your brain's massive jumble of wiring.

When people have cravings, we have found that it is usually because their body has difficulty digesting and absorbing *the foods that are being craved*. For instance, if you have a lot of sugar, it causes your body a lot of distress, yet you will want *more*. Cravings are not an indication that you should give your body more of what you're craving. In fact, the opposite is usually true.

A personal goal that I recommend to people is to have no addictions. This is a mental discipline to the utmost degree. There is no doubt that I enjoy chocolate. But I made it a point that if I am craving chocolate, I avoid it until the craving disappears. This is one example of how you can listen and communicate with your own body.

The Little Voices in Your Head Are Actually Coming From Your Gut

Our gastrointestinal system, when in a healthy state, has approximately one hundred trillion residents known as our gut flora. According to a 2011 research study on nutrients, it is estimated that 90 percent of the cells in our body are microbes.[8] This population is collectively referred to as our microbiome or our gut flora.

Most of these non-human cells are located throughout our gastrointestinal tract, where they provide a natural defense barrier while playing major roles in the making of vitamins, nutrients, and electrolytes. The constant communication of our gut bacteria with your body's cells is the main reason why you can read this book, walk, speak, and every other action your body is able to perform.

The functioning of the microbiome is too complex to be discussed in depth here. We will only briefly review the role of the gut flora in our bodies, but there are numerous books, published by several great authors, that you could read to learn more about this topic.

The important thing to know is that your immunity, nutrient absorption rate, mood, and behavior are strongly influenced by your body's relationship with the bacteria living in your gut. A research study done at UCLA showed an amazing link between brain structure and responses to emotional stimuli. The

---

8 Sender, Ron, et al. "Revised Estimates for the Number of Human and Bacteria Cells in the Body." *Plos Biology*. 19 August 2016. Doi. org/10.1371/journal.pbio.1002533

study looked at the brain's white and gray matter.[9] To keep this simple, the gray matter is the part of the brain that contains nerve cell bodies, and it is where all the action happens. The white matter of the brain is made up of axons, or wires that connect all gray matter areas with areas throughout our body.

The researchers wanted to see how the brain responded while looking at different types of bacteria, specifically the *bacteriodes* and *prevotella* species. The *prevotella* species showed a stronger effect on white areas of the brain that impacted emotions, attention, and sensory processing of various brain regions. The *bacteriodes* species revealed a greater impact on gray matter, affecting areas of the brain like the cerebellum, the frontal regions, and the hippocampus.

In other words, the *bacteriodes* species affected communication between brain regions, just as the Ethernet brings the internet from one area outside our house into our home. The *prevotella* species, in contrast, improved the communication between neurons, just like providing better Wi-Fi or a cable-linking system between a computer and router. This is just a glimpse into how important your microbiome

9 Champeau, Rachel. "Changing gut bacteria through diet affects brain function, UCLA study shows." *UCLA Newsroom*. 28 May 2013. newsroom.ucla.edu/releases/changing-gut-bacteria-through-245617

is to your health, your body's ability to communicate, and your state of mind.

> You and you alone are responsible for listening to your body and determining what it needs and what it doesn't.

Your body's communication system can greatly improve your own ability to heal, sleep, energize, focus, run, and everything else. So many people get into a routine of doing things that put their bodies into a whirlwind; this is what sets up our own disease processes.

Starting today, you can change the rest of your life by simply becoming aware of what your body wants and needs to thrive. So many different aspects of health must be implemented to achieve good health. Communication and awareness are two of the most important aspects that we all need to assess. Making the right changes will help you to build a long, healthy life for yourself.

Having been a pro kick boxer and open style martial arts fighter in my younger years, I have relied on Dr. Weber to put me back together more than once. He has helped me return to mobility many times.

I. Bear
Lead Instructor of Black Dragon Kung Fu
St. Louis, MO

CHAPTER FIVE

Bring It All Together

YOUR BODY REQUIRES REGULAR MAINTENANCE

Just like your car, just like your house, just like every other piece of machinery that you utilize and need to have working in proper order, your body needs maintenance to function at its finest.

Your body never takes a break. It never stops sleeping, it never stops eating, it never stops working for you. When it shows wear and tear, your body is in need of care. Hopefully, in reading this book, you have found some gems that show you when it is necessary to seek care.

Chiropractic Care Is the Best Way to Support the Body's Structural Integrity

Some doctors of chiropractic believe that a simple adjustment to an area that is not moving will create a miraculous change. However, it is not that simple. To understand structural stability, let's look at the basic components of a spinal adjustment.

In Chapter One, we outlined some of the anatomical structures that are important for stability. Now let's explore a little bit deeper.

As we discussed, the joint alarm system called proprioception consists of receptors that govern specific sections of the body. If a muscle is at risk, the proprioceptors fire off a distress signal to the spinal cord, which results in intrinsic muscles guarding movement of individual vertebral segments.

For instance, if you were wrestling with one of your siblings and he happened to bend your fingers backward, this would result in the firing of the proprioceptor system in the joints of your fingers. The system would act to protect your muscles from being overstressed; in our example, the right response could prevent damage to the joints of your hand.

Now let's take that knowledge of defending your joints and apply it to the spine.

If spinal ligaments were damaged via trauma or inflammatory processes, this would cause sensory neurons between your vertebrae to fire a nerve impulse in the muscles surrounding that vertebra. The average person has twenty-four vertebrae in the spine, so you can imagine this process happening at multiple sites.

The muscles that move the spine would try to stabilize the spine; hence, the muscle spasm(s) would occur due to weakening of the ligaments. If the ligaments weaken, the contractile strength of the muscles surrounding each vertebra — including the ones that cover multiple levels along the spine — would increase more and more to maintain stability.

> People in pain are categorized as acute. Those who experience muscle tightness without pain have a chronic issue that is unresolved.

At chiropractic school, we are taught to look for pain mainly in the back, but pain may only be reported by acute or sub-acute patients. Chronic patients will feel stiff and sore while making their first movements of the day, but they often do not report experiencing pain, although the muscle contraction is constant. The skilled chiropractor will recognize this issue and address it accordingly to ensure structural stability is at its best. However, a chiropractor will only be enlisted when you recognize the need for it yourself.

Strong Structural Integrity Means Strong Functionality

As we continue the discussion of structure versus function, let's take a deeper look at how structural imbalances may impact human performance. As doctors of chiropractic, we know that *everything can affect everything*.

To illustrate this, let's look at someone who has flat feet, otherwise known as *hyperpronation*. This condition results in an inward torsion in the lower limbs. This torsion starts at the pelvis and torques downward in a spiral pattern that results in muscle fatigue and over-stretched ligaments in the foot causing the arch to flatten or fall.

The attachment site for the head of the femur is in the hip joint, which—up to this point in time—is still balanced. However, as the inside foot bones or metatarsals fall toward the ground along with the tibia, as the lower joints spiral downward and the pelvis goes the opposite way, this causes a major shearing force at the knee joint.

In times of trauma, falls, or repeated intense activities, this shearing may cause your knee meniscus, anterior cruciate ligament (ACL), or posterior cruciate ligament (PCL) to tear. Even if a person is lucky enough not to cause trauma to their knee, the torsion of the leg will eventually continue up to impact the pelvis, causing a pelvic imbalance, also known as a sacroiliac subluxation, like the situation we discussed in Chapter One.

We began this illustration with a person who had symptoms from flat feet, which subsequently caused knee injury and a severe pelvic imbalance. You can see how one imbalance can cause a chain of structural consequences. This is why we say *everything can affect everything*.

We can easily take this illustration further. I cannot emphasize the significance of the pelvic anatomy enough. It has an impact on human physiology in many ways, and imbalances can affect other body systems.

For example, according to a research article in 2015 from *Biological Sciences*, the ability to regulate body temperature is affected by the width and the depth of the pelvic floor, which plays a crucial role in determining overall body proportions.[10]

For most individuals, the structural stability of our biomechanical system relies on the stability of the

---

10 Gruss, Laura Tobias, and Daniel Schmitt. "The evolution of the human pelvis: changing adaptations to bipedalism, obstetrics and thermoregulation." *The Royal Society*. 05 March 2015. doi.org/10.1098/rstb.2014.0063

pelvis. It is the practitioner's responsibility to make sure the joints above and below the pelvis are able to work together as one unit. This allows the muscles to contract fully, which gives us our full strength. Most importantly, pelvic stability is required to allow proper fluid flow to and from our limbs. People who suffer from flat feet are often knock-kneed, which leads to decreased muscle strength and fluid circulation compared to those whose legs and pelvis are balanced.

Body Communication Depends on the Structural Integrity of Its Systems

So many people in today's society believe that hormones are solely to blame for symptoms like low energy levels, poor sleep quality, and an inability to stay on task. As we discussed previously, it is never just one thing; it is everything at once. Our bodies are made up of millions of cells that are all designed to work as one unit.

Transport and communication are vital parts of this process. It is the sole job of our blood to bring proper oxygenation to cells, hormones to receptor sites, and immune cells to areas needed to fight off infections or tissues in need of healing. It is critical that our blood flow be adequate and efficient to deliver the necessary components to our cells.

What system orchestrates this?

You may have guessed it is your autonomic nervous system, and you wouldn't be wrong. But your autonomic nervous system answers to an even higher force known as *innate intelligence*. Innate intelligence is recognized across multiple fields of medicine, especially alternative medicine. Your innate intelligence originated with the miraculous union of your mother's egg and your father's sperm to make the first pair of cells that made you. This amazing system is our body's way of orchestrating nerves, cells, organs, and everything else that makes you and me.

My main point is to make it clear that if your body's structural system loses its integrity, then its best way of communication is impaired. Your overall function would be drastically lowered, leading to fatigue, allergies, weight gain, insomnia, and nearly every other sign or symptom you have heard, read, or felt. It is of critical importance that everybody makes sure their body's biomechanical structure is of the very best integrity to ensure the best health and nutrition for each cell.

Hopefully, this information helps to open you to the possibility in your mind that your body does need maintenance in all ways, shapes, and forms.

Chiropractic is not the only method, but it is the only one that truly deals with the structural stressors of daily life. Alternative forms of therapy, like massage, acupuncture, Bowen therapy, and numerous others, are extremely beneficial, and I do not wish to take anything away from them. But they don't do what the chiropractic adjustment does to help heal our bodies.

YOUR BODY IS ONLY AS GOOD AS THE CARE YOU GIVE IT

Throughout the book, we have discussed all the aspects that can harm and cause dis-ease to our body, but it is also critical to understand the care your body requires and the best ways to go about it. Let's explore that now.

If You Don't Care, Your Body Won't Care

We tend to assume that our bodies will just keep on going.

What happens if I don't exercise this week?

What happens to me if I eat fast food tomorrow?

We can ask all the *what if* questions we want, but the answer will still be the same. We'll do what we can with what we have to work with. Our bodies are programmed to live on whatever resources are available. Although many people understand this, few rarely ever take the necessary action to better their scenario.

Why don't we act to better our health?

Among the more common excuses are:

- *I don't have time.*
- *I'm not sure what I should be doing.*
- *How do I know this is the right thing for me?*

Hopefully, reading this book has helped you begin to find some answers. If not, if you would like some help finding the answers to your situation, you are welcome to contact our office through our website at www.quantumchiroca.com.

The bottom line is the title of this section: *If you don't care, neither does the body.* Your body will not take care of itself. If you don't care for it, it will try to keep going the best it can. If you step up, your body will respond.

How can you begin?

Let's start with nutrition and exercise.

Better Nutrition = Better Quality of Life

If you are following the seasons at your local farmer's market, you are seeing the vast array of food available to you.

It is only by eating a wide variety of vegetables and fruits that you will get the necessary vitamins, minerals, and co-factors needed to support processes like detoxification, digestion, absorption, circulation, and healing. If you choose a life of fast, processed, or sugary type foods even though you know they are bad for you, you will be digging yourself into a hole, and you will eventually have to contend with the consequences. You will need to make healthy changes to have the quality of life you want to live.

Nutritional supplements are a great way to get loads of nutrition in a small space. Look carefully at the ingredients: the fewer fillers, the better. When you buy a supplement from a store like Wal-Mart or GNC, it is typically poorer quality than the supplements received from doctor's offices like ours. Our supplements are tested, researched, and tested again for cleanliness and purity, and they are guaranteed to be the best support for you and your path to wellness.

It is well-known that in today's society there is a massive epidemic of childhood obesity, ADD, ADHD, and dementia. Cancer cases are skyrocketing far higher than ever before. This is not because our society doesn't care about people. It's because the marketing teams that sell sugar, soda, and all the other items we know are not beneficial to us don't care about your quality of life, only the levels of their profit margins.

Do you have a family to provide nutrition for, but aren't sure how to go about it?

The best thing you can do for you and your family is to take one step at a time to make the right choices to better your health. Just remember what the flight crew tells you when you are getting ready for takeoff: in emergencies, you should *put your mask on first, then help your child.*

Why is this, you think?

Simple. Before you can help them, you have to be well yourself. You have to care about yourself enough to make sure they are taking care of themselves as well. Take care of yourself, and set a good example for your family members. One day, your children will thank you for being health-conscious.

More Motion = Healthier Body

Most adults are aware that they need to exercise in some way, shape, or form. Moderate activity, as discussed previously, is one of the best ways to ensure that your body is not exceeding its physiological limits. Let's bring the topic of child's play to this. Most adults joke that they wish they could bottle their child's energy into a bottle for themselves. These days, however, we are beginning to see a new era in which kids are more sedentary than ever before.

In 2016, Canadian studies found that 62 percent of children between the ages of two and four and 26 percent of children under the age of thirteen did not meet recommended activity levels, but exceeded their recommended screen time for activities like gaming and TV. This lack of physical activity is a very strong promoter of chronic diseases, including cardiovascular disease, type 2 diabetes, and osteoporosis, as well as an overall diminished IQ and a lowered ability to socialize with others.[11]

Our bodies are made to move.

The moral of the story is our bodies are made to move. From the time we learn to crawl, we are moving. At our office, we encourage motion in every form possible, whether it is swimming, running, dancing, or martial arts. Anything you enjoy is fine. The more

11 Barnes, Joel D., Christine Cameron, et. al. "Results from Canada's ParticipACTION Report Card on Physical Activity for Children and Youth." doi: org/10.1123/jpah.2016-0300

you enjoy the activity, the more you will be willing to spend time doing it.

As we've discussed previously in multiple chapters, you create your own health. You have more control over your health than you realize. You are the one who sets the bar on what you can and cannot do. No matter what specific efforts you are making for your health, don't stop; always move forward.

We Have an Adult Nervous System by the Age of Seven

Would you be surprised to discover that the habits we learned at a young age have an impact on our lives as adults?

I am sure most of you are not too surprised by this because you have seen it to be true. Our relationships with our parents, our household environment, and our behaviors growing up become factors in our ability to handle stress, relationships, and many other issues in our adult lives. The topic of childhood development alone could be a book in itself — and there are already several out there — but let me touch on a few items in this area just the same.

The first item is breastfeeding. James W. Anderson, a professor of medicine and clinical nutrition at the University of Kentucky in Lexington, reported in the *American Journal of Clinical Nutrition* in October 1999 that suckled infants averaged three to five points higher in IQ than formula-fed babies.[12] What was more impressive was that the longer the infant breastfed, the greater the gain in IQ points. Over nine months of breastfeeding, the effects appeared to end. Another study out of the University of Kentucky pointed out that increased IQ could be attributed to the enhanced bonding between the mother and the nursing infant, where it was less pronounced in mothers who formula-fed their kids.[13] Breastfeeding is nothing but great for building a healthy brain for a growing youngster.

The second point is about early brain growth. During our critical years of development between the ages of one and three, this period of brain growth in the infant has twice as many neurons and twice as many synapses, which are gap junctions between neurons that allow neurotransmitters to send signals, versus adults. It is critical during these years that the infant be nurtured. Research has established that touching and stroking are essential for a healthy development, as

---

12 Anderson, James W., Bryan M. Johnstone, and Daniel T. Remley. "Breast-feeding and cognitive development: a meta-analysis." The American Journal of Clinical Nutrition. 01 October, 1999. Doi: org/10.109/ajcn/70.4.525
13 "Kentucky Study Shows Breast-Feeding Increases Babies' IQ." Science Daily. 28 September, 1999. sciencedaily.com/ releases/1999/09/990928075022.htm

well as normal nerve growth. A study done by Mark Spit of the Dupont Research Laboratories found that laboratory animal infants deprived of their mother's care lost brain cells at twice the rate compared to those who were cared for by their moms.[14] The study found that stroking stimulates the production of chemicals that inhibit stress hormones like cortisol, which harm brain cells.

A major epidemic that is being discussed among researchers today is the effect of screen time on young brains. The amount of time watching TV and gaming, to name a few activities, has negative impacts on developing nervous systems. The use of electronics such as cell phones and TVs should be limited so that the child has enough time to play, sleep, talk, and study. More recent studies are beginning to link amounts of screen use to anxiety, depression, excessive tantrums, short-term memory losses, ADD, ADHD, some types of behavior, poor self-relation, and social immaturity.

Being a parent is a full-time job, and I give praise to every parent who does their best every day to create a loving, positive environment for all the youngsters in their care. Please remember that your kids learn

14 Hotz, Robert Lee. "Neglect Harms Infants' Brains, Researchers Say." *Los Angeles Times*. 28 October 1997. articles.latimes.com/1997/oct/28/news/mn-47555

behaviors by what they see and feel. If change is necessary for a healthier lifestyle, be sure to change the environment in which the family interacts for a long-lasting benefit. Just remember that kids will become adults, so all the information in this book rings true for them as well, including structural and functional health.

HEALTHY BODY, HEALTHY MIND, STRONG SPIRIT

The biomechanical system is just one aspect of our health that we need to consider. It is becoming better understood that emotional and mental health are also important. Those who have invested the time also know that the spiritual aspect of our being is highly critical. I won't talk too much about the spiritual aspect, but our spiritual health is impacted by both mind and body.

You Are What You Eat

What you eat today is walking and talking tomorrow.

~ Jack LaLanne

This quote is true on so many levels. A friend in high school would designate a day during the week when he would binge eat because, during the other six days, he was on a strict eating schedule for his weight lifting. Looking back at it now, we can honestly say this was not the best way to go about it.

Years later, when starting my practice, my knowledge of nutrition and wellness rose sharply because I learned that what I had been taught as a student and well before chiropractic college was fake news.

For instance, did you know breads and whole grains are not good for you?

The spike in the blood sugar that we get from breads isn't healthy, but this isn't the most severe problem. It is the whole grain. In the whole of the grain are high amounts of lectins, otherwise known as nature's poison. Lectins are very dangerous in that they resist digestion and are extremely dangerous to our gut flora by shifting the balance of the good and bad bacteria. One of the worst culprits is wheat germ gluten, which is found in wheat and other seeds. If this topic interests you, I highly recommend reading Dr. Steven Gundry's 2017 book, *The Plant Paradox: The Hidden Dangers in "Healthy" Foods that Cause Disease and Weight Gain* and Dr. David Peterson's 2013 book, *Lectin Free Diet: A Patient Resource Guide to Edible Enemies.*

Considering lectins and gut flora, our office recommends the following:

1. Eat according to the seasons.
2. Eat according to the rainbow.
3. Eat fermented foods.

Eat according to the season, when fruits and vegetables are at their peak ripeness. Lectins are in everything derived from plant life, and our goal is to keep them low. Eating according to the season almost always allows your lectin quality to be low because lectins are high in foods that are not fully ripened. This deters predators from eating before the seeds are ready to start a new generation of growth. Often the color of the fruit changes when it is fully ripe. For example, most apples are green when they are developing, but when they are ripe, they turn a dark red and catch your eye as you are walking through the orchard.

Next, *eat according to the rainbow.* If you always eat multiple colors, this ensures you are eating a variety of fruit and vegetables, all of which are extremely beneficial to your gut flora. By eating different foods throughout the week and every other week, you are creating a diverse gut flora. A lack of gut flora can lead to allergies, eczema, acne, leaky gut issues, migraines, autoimmunity, and more. Eat according to the rainbow to avoid those gloomy days of ill health.

Last, but not least, *eat fermented foods.*

What are fermented foods, you ask?

The fermentation process is the conversion of carbohydrates to alcohol and organic acids, using microbes such as yeast and bacterial strains under a low-oxygen environment. Foods like yogurt, sauerkraut, kimchi, and pickles are just a few examples of well-known fermented foods. These types of food introduce live strains of bacteria to our gut daily, which improves immunity and cell-to-cell communication. Fermented foods are very good for you and are easy to make.

Healthy eating is a key component to improving your condition, as well as prolonging your life. You ask any athlete, weight lifter, actor, or anyone else who actively tries to stay in good shape: good performance and physique are not possible without a great meal plan. Make eating right the most important part of your recipe for long-lasting health.

You Are What You Think

Psychology is field of study that extends deeply into so many different areas that it can be overwhelming. Great authors like Napoleon Hill discuss in much detail the term *auto-suggestion*. Psychiatrists like Dr. David Hawkins break down the science and frequency of specific emotions. Dr. Joe Dispenza and Dr. Bruce Lipton break down the cellular components of how our thoughts and beliefs affect our biochemistry and how they are directly connected to our emotions and internal stressors. All these authors are pioneers in the understanding of our thoughts and intentions.

It is my goal to keep this simple. In every movie I watched as a kid, there was a villain and a hero, a good guy and a bad guy. Let's use this analogy. The good guy is always trying to upset the balance by hurting, lying, or breaking apart what the other guy is trying to save and keep together. Let's give these two characters names. We'll call them *love* and *hate*.

Hate despises everything about everyone and wants nothing to grow or be together. Love is the No. 1 most powerful emotion known to humans. It brings everyone together. When one of these two emotion dominates our thoughts, it can be a critical turning point in our health.

For instance, think of that one individual who is always happy and loves to see you. This person doesn't have anything negative to say about anyone. You know that person is full of love, and it's contagious. Now think of that individual who has nothing good to say about anyone or anything, who loves to blame, shame, or justify his or her actions in every scenario.

Which individual would you want to spend time with?

When our thoughts are pure, our health is on the right track. In a previous chapter, we discussed mental discipline. It is important to keep striving, even though we all fall now and then. We are human. It is our duty to be contributing members to our community and to inspire love and health in one another. When we can love and praise our bodies for what we were given, our health and vitality are more likely to return in abundance.

For those who enjoy affirmations, please use these to help change your thoughts about yourself:

- *I purge my body of all dark thoughts that hold back my true healing.*

- *I know now that anything I picture in my mind will be amplified in my own health.*

- *I will use this power only to see good things. I love and praise my body for all that I am.*

Taking Care of You

What makes your world?

Take a second and think of those individuals who depend on you.

Is it your spouse, your parents, your kid, your boss, your employees?

Have you put yourself on your list?

Look at your list. Hopefully, you will see how important your life is to everyone in your world. If you have put yourself last on your list of people who need help, read this book again. Making sure you are healthy guarantees that those around you will be healthy because you will be there to make sure they are getting the correct care they need.

Keep your structure strong through chiropractic care, eat the colors of the rainbow while in season to ensure a healthy gut microbiome and lower your risk of poisonous toxins by lowering your lectin intake. Get regular exercise throughout your week to support a strong body and mind, and in doing so, you will support a strong spirit through determination and perseverance.

We recommend everyone get lab testing done at least once a year to make sure that there are no unpleasant surprises in the near future. The bottom line is, as you strive to make healthy life habits, you need to be reassured that what you are doing is working for you. So, please consult your doctor and have them run the appropriate tests for you.

The last item I would like to share with you before closing this chapter speaks to the manner in which you heal yourself. In healing one's self, we must come together. When our bodies are in a state of hate or inflammation, our bodies are feeling apart. It is only by coming together that we can keep away from ill health.

When you eat foods that are not beneficial to you, it tears your cells apart through the process of inflammation. When we hate ourselves, it tears us apart both emotionally and physically. When you use the emotion of love in your daily life, it becomes a part of your body, mind, and spirit, which is the greatest therapy that anyone can give another. This is the practice of art and healing we use at Quantum Chiropractic, and we hope to promote this practice and inspire others to use it to find good health.

I've gone to a couple of chiropractors before, and some acute issues were addressed. But then I came across Jim and Pauline Weber, who are SOT® chiropractors. I was really excited to meet them and see how their treatments would be. In my initial consultation, Dr. Jim assessed the structural setup of my entire body.

He completed various assessments from different Chiropractic approaches, including assessing the body's weakness patterns. Dr. Jim tested my reflexes, balance, and strength at various times, some based on the initial issues I expressed.

I never go in feeling like I'm just being put through the motions. I can physically and visually notice the difference when something has been fixed that I didn't even realize was wrong.

Outside of his professional techniques and experience, Dr. Jim is a friendly and a personable person, which makes seeing him a great experience overall.

J. Head
Sacramento, CA

Conclusion

This book is only a peek into the world of structural and functional health care.

After reading this book, we hope you have come to the same conclusions we have:

For the best structural and functional performance of our bodies, we must have a balanced pelvis and cranium and a properly functioning autonomic nervous system that comes from a balanced spine and all its incoming data from organs and tissues — muscles, ligaments, etc.

- Inflammation and stress must be reduced to allow for the best blood flow, oxygenation of tissues, and cellular communications. For example, immune cells, hormones, neurotransmitters, etc.

- Eating healthfully is a choice as well as a lifestyle. Just remember that we only have one life to live, and how we take care of it today allows us to be happy tomorrow.

- Chiropractic is an underutilized tool that helps bring happiness and joy to millions around the world.

Trying to achieve health without chiropractic is like:

- A drawer that is not on its track. It will close — just not easily or straight.

- Trying to determine your maximum weight on a bench without a spotter. The spotter, just like the chiropractor, is assisting you to reach your fullest potential at that moment.

- A sliding screen door. When it is off its track, it will still close but with much more effort. When the screen door is on the track, it moves effortlessly.

- A consistent workout routine. Keeping up around the house is just like chiropractic maintenance care that keeps you stronger and healthier for life.

Chiropractic is the art of increasing efficiency in our bodies moving parts. The majority of patients who leave our office after the first visit comment that they are out of pain but they feel *lighter*. It is not that they have lost weight, but their body does not have to work so hard to stand up.

Please keep in mind that no one in this world is going to take better care of you than you. The decision to live a happy, healthier life must start with the decision to strive for a healthier lifestyle. We are all human and make mistakes. Don't beat yourself up when you fall, when you eat the wrong thing, or do something else unhealthy. Learn from your mistakes so you don't make them again. Stressing about what you did only leads to more stress and frustration. Be happy that you recognize the error, correct what you are able to, and keep striving for a happier, healthier life. Today is a brand new day.

> *A journey of a thousand miles begins with a single step.*
>
> ~ Bao Su

Hopefully, this book has opened your eyes to the possibility that anything can cause anything. The body is a solitary unit with trillions of cells and even more microbes working together for the greater good of your health. Both chiropractic care and gut-related issues are highly overlooked in today's society. Most people have no clue that their headaches, migraines, eczema, autoimmune disease, ADD, ADHD, fibromyalgia, and other conditions are being stimulated by an underlying gut issue. Nutritional imbalances may be expressed by the body as muscle soreness and tightness, and as they continue unaddressed, the disease process begins.

The importance of a vast number of nutrition-related issues is drastically underestimated. Eating healthy food is a choice as well as a lifestyle. Just remember that we only have one life to live, and how we take care of it today allows us to be happy tomorrow.

There are probably millions of medical textbooks and other health-related books that can describe the ailments that patients might experience. However, rarely do we ever have patients whom we can treat as simply as reading a cookbook. More often than not, people are a combination of several factors that impede their health in some way, shape, or form. This is why it's great to learn and research, but please don't diagnose yourself without discussing it with your doctor first.

As we have discussed in previous chapters, your mind is a powerful factor in your health. If you decide that you have a particular issue, your mind has already sent a stress signal throughout your body, which creates a whole host of issues that subconsciously you have programmed to work against you, to create more internal stress.

Chiropractic is a field of medicine that is gaining recognition and acceptance among our peers in the medical profession. Not every chiropractor is the same. Not everyone is going to work well with you.

Find the doctor who listens to you and acknowledges you for who you are and what you are going through.

At Quantum Chiropractic, we specialize in dealing with chronic pain. If you have a case you would like us to look at, you can reach us through our website, quantumchiroca.com, or check us out on Facebook at facebook.com/quantumchiroca. We would love to hear your stories and thoughts about the information in this book. Please keep in touch.

Our staff at Quantum Chiropractic in Sacramento, California, has had years of relentless training and is constantly striving to make sure patients get everything they want plus more. We believe that when a person has their health, they can live, dream, and make memories that will be cherished for years to come. Best wishes to you.

Next Steps

It is clear to me that those who want help will go to the end of the world to find it. Hopefully, this book is instrumental in that pursuit to finding a solution for those who need it.

This book is designed for everyday people and healthcare practitioners alike. It is my goal to get information out there so chiropractic is not viewed with skepticism anymore. In the past, chiropractic was poorly understood and laughed at by other health care providers but now, with new technology and a better understanding of anatomy and physiology, we can be sure of what we are accomplishing.

Our office motto is *Science Guided Care for Natural Healing*. We aim to do just that.

You are welcome to contact our office. If you would like our input on a health concern, please do not hesitate to call or email. We have patients all over the United States.

Our contact information is on our website: quantumchiroca.com.

You can also contact us through our Facebook page: QuantumChiroCA.

You may contact our office directly at 916-616-1595.

About the Author

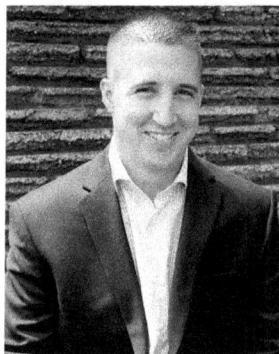

Dr. James Weber is a sacro-occipital chiropractor who has advanced training and certifications in internal health, craniopathy, and pediatrics. While starting out in practice, he recognized that the healing art of chiropractic is powerful; however, it's only part of the equation. The rest is establishing healthy habits that influence the mind, body, and spirit.

Dr. James Weber graduated Logan College of Chiropractic in August 2009 with his bachelors in human biology and his doctorate of chiropractic. He was introduced to several great doctors who inspired him to look outside the traditional chiropractic model. Within two years of beginning his practice, other healthcare practitioners were consulting with him on cases around the country. When Dr. Weber is not in the office, he is often attending seminars to educate his clients, or he is educating other doctors.

Dr. Weber is not your typical "whack & crack" chiropractor. He realizes your time is precious, and it should not be spent in ill health. His team at Quantum Chiropractic offers a comprehensive approach to health and wellness. At our office, our team will take an in-depth look at what your body is going through while taking a thorough assessment of your signs and symptoms. Tie that all together with laboratory testing, and you have a comprehensive evaluation of the stressors your body is facing.